Eating Right for
Type 2 Diabetes

Eating Right for Type 2 Diabetes

✦

A Christian Perspective on a Traumatic Disease

Desmond Ford, PhD

iUniverse, Inc.
New York Lincoln Shanghai

Eating Right for Type 2 Diabetes
A Christian Perspective on a Traumatic Disease

iUniverse, Inc.

For information address:
iUniverse, Inc.
2021 Pine Lake Road, Suite 100
Lincoln, NE 68512
www.iuniverse.com

ISBN: 0-595-32779-6

Printed in the United States of America

This book is intended to be a practical help to the diabetic but it is not a comprehensive guide. Its counsels should be studied in conjunction with regular consultations with a specialist in diabetes.

This book and others by Desmond Ford are available
In the USA from:
www.goodnewsunlimited.org
E-mail: gnu@goodnewsunlimited.org

In Canada, contact:
www.goodnewsunlimited.org/canada.cfm

In Australia, contact: Book Order Department, GNU,
P.O. Box 6788, Unit 2, 54-60 Industry Drive,
Tweed Heads South, N.S.W. 2486, Australia.
Price, including postage and handling = $30.00 (Australian)
www.goodnewsunlimited.org.au.
e-mail: carolyn@goodnewsunlimited.org.au

To find out more about Dr. Desmond Ford,
visit his website at www.desford.org.au.

Dedicated to Marion Fritz—a woman who didn't need this book, but who was my friend and faithful fellow minister in fulfilling the Great Commission for more than two decades.

Contents

Quotable Quotes

You, the individual, can do more for your own health and well being than any doctor, any hospital and drug, any exotic medical advice.

—C. Everett Koop, M.D., Former Surgeon General of the U.S.

Diabetes is probably the pleasantest of all chronic diseases. It is not painful, disfiguring, depressing, contagious or otherwise devastating—if recognized and kept under control.

—Justin J. Schifferer, *Family Medical Encyclopedia*, p. 117.

I feel very positive about my "malfunction" [diabetes]. It means that...I exercise more than most people, watch my diet more than most people, and as a consequence, I think I am healthier than most people.

—Mary Tyler Moore

Disgusted at having to listen to this tired old litany of the supposedly inevitable dire consequence of diabetes, June glanced over at diabetic triathelete Bill Carlson, who was seated in the audience near us. He was lean, fit, and glowing with health. He'd been on a bike ride of a hundred and ten miles the day before and on his usual long-distance run that very morning. What have those statistics to do with him?

June thought about herself and the fact that, at her age (mid-60s), she was healthier and in much better shape than all of her non-diabetic contemporaries and even many women ten or fifteen years younger. What do these statistics have to do with her? After twenty-five years of diabetes, she had zero diabetes complications.

—Peter A. Lodewick, M.D., June Biermann, and Barbara Toohey,
The Diabetic Man, pp. 13-14.

Despite all the diabetics among us (one out of four Americans is an actual or potential diabetic, or a "carrier"—and the incidence is increasing by almost 10 percent every year), there are still a great many popular and important misconceptions about this disorder.

—I. Rosenfeld, *Second Opinion,* p. 56.

I don't like having diabetes; I hate it. But somehow it has forced me to learn how to take care of myself. I wouldn't give up knowing how to do that for anything in the world.

—Peter A. Lodewick, M.D., June Biermann, and Barbara Toohey,
The Diabetic Man, p. 314.

Foreword

Everything eventually wears out, and our bodies are no exception. Indeed, degenerative disorders are posed to be the scourge of the 21st century. At the turn of the 20th century, there were no effective treatments for infectious diseases. Now that we have, at least for now, overcome such curses, it is disorders that result from gradual wearing out and breaking down that keep us conscious of the fact that God alone is immortal.

Some of the physical wear and tear is accelerated by our own habits, but sometimes by inheritance and, at other times, for no apparent reason. Sometimes one part of our body wears out much faster than other parts. Because of this, someone who has lived an exemplary healthy life can still end up with a pancreas that gives up when the rest of the body is still strong and vigorous. Dr. Desmond Ford who has set an example in healthy living now explains his personal experience with diabetes. The disorder in his case is not due to either overnutrition or underactivity, two factors that help explain diabetes in many individuals.

Dr. Ford has also been a spiritual beacon pointing tens of thousands to God's grace. Who better then to help others come to terms with "a thorn in the flesh, a messenger from Satan" (2 Cor 12:7), to remind us that we are human, and God is God. Dr. Ford does not stop there, however. He proceeds to discuss his own attempts to control his glucose levels with what he chooses to call the "high road of diet and exercise." Actually there is no "low road," since all those with diabetes need to be careful with their eating. Admittedly, pharmacology makes the burden lighter for many individuals. On the other hand, if the pancreas is severely depleted of insulin there simply is no diet that will help. The Nobel Prize for the discovery of insulin, the lifesaver of tens of thousands with severe insulin lack, attests to that.

Dr. Ford's efforts here are not a technical review of either diabetes or nutrition. There is simply a vast amount of scientific research on the topic, and the interested person needs to look elsewhere for such a scientific analysis. This work presents Dr. Ford's experience, and others can benefit from that.

Stephen Lillioja
M.B., Ch.B., F.R.A.C.P.,
Associate Professor of Medicine
University of New South Wales, Australia.

As a practicing physician, I have been interested in life-style and its effects on health for some four decades. I have read Dr. Desmond Ford's manuscript with interest and have no hesitation in recommending it for serious consideration by all Type 2 diabetics. Its concepts are in accord with our modern understanding of this puzzling, but increasingly common condition.

Alan A. Jones, M.D., orthopedic surgeon
M.B., B.S. (Sydney), F.R.C.S. (Edin.), M.A.C.N.E.M.

Acknowledgements

I would like to thank Molly Brown of Good News Unlimited, California, U.S.A., and Lauren Grieve my daughter's secretary, for typing the original manuscript, and my wife Gill for preparing the manuscript for publication. I appreciate those who helped by reading the manuscript, particularly Dr. Stephen Lillioja, a diabetes specialist in Sydney, Australia, and Dr. Alan Jones, an orthopedic surgeon in Coffs Harbour, Australia.

A Personal Note to My Readers

Apart from childhood diphtheria, I have had seventy-five years of excellent health. This is despite sixty-five years of daily, intense application to books, the demands of teaching and writing, and decades of frequent travel on speaking itineraries with all the inevitable stresses. Even now, I have no overt symptoms of illness. But since a traumatic accident in Russia, I have had type 2 diabetes.

That discovery led me to ransack libraries in several countries for all relevant medical knowledge about type 2 diabetes—the third cause of death in the Western world.

Learning that all diabetic drugs can have serious side effects, I resolved to avoid their use for as long as possible. This meant dramatic changes in my eating habits. Before, as a vegetarian for over half a century, I ate a diet largely made up of fruit, vegetables, nuts, legumes, and whole grains. Now I had to change what many experts acknowledge is the ideal diet for most people. Why? Because the advocates of the cutting edge of modern diabetic therapy now warn against the traditional high carbohydrate diet recommended for diabetics. This was introduced after finding out that the early diabetics on low carbohydrate diets were consuming a lot of animal products and dying prematurely of heart disease.

The present emphasis by top researchers is to replace grains and other high-carbohydrate-containing foods with monounsaturates (avocados, olives, soybeans, nuts, flax, and sesame seeds, etc.), plus a generous partaking of raw salad, lightly cooked vegetables, and some eggs and cheese.

Accompanying the dietary recommendations is the advice (long known and taught) that exercise at the right time and in the right amount acts like insulin for many diabetics.

Now, for years, I have pursued this regimen and found it to work very well. I use neither insulin nor oral medications and never experience the episodes of hypoglycemia, which regularly attend the traditional therapies. Most days, I jog, walk, and swim or cycle, covering about 10 miles by foot. My work program absorbs about fifty hours per week.

I add a caution that there are unique differences among people with diabetes. Some people, particularly type 1 diabetics, cannot manage diabetes by food control alone. They have to take medication. Nonetheless, every diabetic needs to scrupulously attend to diet. So the suggestions in this book remain pertinent for them.

I would have paid big money to have owned this book when I first learned I had diabetes. May its practical counsels and Christian insights be a means of alleviating the physical, mental, and emotional trauma of every diabetic reader.

Wishing you great health,

Desmond Ford

3 John 2: "My heartfelt prayer for you, my dear friend, is that you may be as healthy and prosperous in every way as you are in soul." J. B. Phillip's Translation.

Postscript

Since finishing this book some time ago I have continued to research the subject and conducted hundreds of experiments on myself with blood sugar measurements, a diet chronicle and noting the impact of exercise. The results confirm what I have previously written, but I have become convinced that a few points need added emphasis in order to give the most practical help possible.

The most recent pronouncements of the ADA and many endocrinologists affirm that a high carbohydrate diet should be avoided, and monounsaturates and salad vegetables should replace them—in other words such foods as avocados, raw nuts, olives, linseed (flaxseed), sesame seeds, sunflower seeds, pepitas, soybeans, and greens, for example lettuce, spinach, celery, parsley, eggplant, and zucchinis.

It has also become increasingly apparent that the control of blood pressure is as or more important than the control of blood sugar levels. This is best achieved by diet and exercise, not drugs. All drugs, without exception, have some negative result on health, though there is certainly a place for drugs for people unable to control their life-style (or with diabetes that does not respond to such controls). The only difference between a drug and a poison is the dose. The nearer one gets to a vegetarian diet, usually the lower the blood pressure.

Because there are scores or even hundreds of shocks and disappointments when regularly using a blood sugar monitor, one clear fact should be kept in mind. This fact particularly applies to those using the therapies of diet and physical activity alone, but it has relevance for all diabetics. At this point in time medical science has no therapy that can exactly control blood glucose. Thus practically all diabetics on insulin or diabetic pills have recurring hypoglycemic attacks. These can be dangerous, particularly for the elderly and those who sleep on their own. The young can handle "hypos" usually with little lasting damage, but it is not so for those advanced in years.

The majority of type 2 diabetics are in this category. In view of this, the most recent expert pronouncements counsel that it is preferable to have one's blood sugar somewhat high, rather than risk "hypos." There is only slight practical difference as regards complications for those with an HBA1C of 8 compared to

<u>those under intensive therapy who have a measurement of 7. Please read that</u> <u>again—it is most important.</u>

If you are now past your fifties you risk brain damage if you suffer recurring "hypos." And, as mentioned, if you live and sleep alone the risk is intensified. Therefore, when most discouraged by the monitor results remind yourself that the use (or greater use) of insulin or pills as the available option will not save you from inevitable (for most) higher levels. This is not a plea for carelessness or indulgence but a reminder that hypoglycemic attacks for the elderly can do more harm than temporary rises in blood glucose.

Observe the word "temporary" in the last sentence. The thing to do in such instances is to go out and walk. For most people a brisk walk reduces the numbers by one per minute, or two if you jog.

For most of us (breaking the usual dietetic rule), breakfast should have the least calories. But it need not be unsatisfying if nuts and/or avocados are included. It is of great practical importance to remember that, while carbohydrates eaten (or drunk) by themselves result in meteoric rises in blood sugar, a small use of the same when preceded (best) or accompanied by <u>fat and/or protein</u> <u>slows down such rises</u>. Don't miss this: <u>the juice of one or two sizeable lemons</u> <u>will contribute to the same result</u>.

(The section on diabetes in the latest edition of Lange's *Current Medical Diagnosis and Treatment, 2004* is invaluable, and worthy of very close study.)

There is no substitute for discipline for the diabetic (including those on insulin). This is the one disease where the patient determines 99 percent of the outcome. Here the Christian has a tremendous advantage, for we know not only that our bodies are the temple of God, but also that the Holy Spirit is willing to motivate and strengthen us for our continuing battles. Read often Psalm 23; Romans 8:28-39; Phil 4:4-13.

Sursum Corda (lift up your hearts!)

Introduction

There are approximately eight million Christian diabetics in the USA, and every year another quarter million churchgoers are diagnosed as victims of this malady. The medical verdict is no light one, for every year diabetic complications include 55,000 lower extremity problems or amputations, over 13,000 cases of end-stage renal disease, 15,000 new cases of blindness, and 2.7 million hospitalizations. Diabetes is increasing at the rate of 10 percent per year, and it is now the third cause of death.

But why a book addressed to Christian diabetics? Aren't all diabetics the same? Emphatically they are not! You might as well inquire whether there is any difference between a prince and a pauper or a giant and a pygmy.

God loves every individual on the planet, whether they acknowledge him or not. But he has a covenant relationship with those who know Christ as Savior and Lord. They no longer live on their own or by their own resources. They have all heaven backing them and all the wealth of omnipotence and omniscience.

Furthermore, all endocrinologists are agreed that the diabetic, to a large extent, must be his or her own doctor, inasmuch as the individual patient manages the treatment daily.

Here is where Christians in many cases have a tremendous advantage. It is impossible to be a mature Christian without having learned through grace the duty, privilege, and blessing of discipline. See 1 Corinthians 9:24-27 and observe the last item in the list of the fruits of the Spirit—the climactic virtue of self-control. Above all other factors, discipline is the condition for diabetic wellbeing.

Denial, anger, and despair are typical responses to the bad news that one has become a diabetic. But the Christian can say with Christ, "The Father hath not left me alone." All heaven is on our side and at our side. "We know that ALL things work together for good to them that love God." We also remember the words of our Lord: "What I do thou knowest not now, but thou shalt know hereafter" (Jn 13:7).

In this small book, the Christian view of stress and tragedy will be spelled out. Robert Louis Stevenson used to say that what matters is not the hand you have been dealt, but how you play it. He was right, and the experience of every mature believer testifies to that liberating fact.

There is another plus for the Christian. He recognizes the body as the temple of God, and this recognition supplies the motivation for discipline in all the habits of life. While this book offers the most recent medical insights for managing diabetes successfully, the counsel will only help those who know that "all things are possible to him that believeth," and that God is ready and willing to supply our every need through his riches in glory. (See Philippians 4:19.) Others will blanch at the prospect of unending discipline all the days of their lives.

Even Christians are dependent to a large degree on the truths medical science can offer, and in this tiny volume will be found the answers to many of the most pressing questions all newly diagnosed diabetics ask. For those who wish to be the best possible stewards of their health and opportunities, this knowledge is worth more than a fortune.

I do not write as a spectator of the medical scene. I have diabetes myself and know firsthand the shock, the alarm, and the bewilderment of receiving that diagnosis. I have two research Ph.D.s, and I have spent hundreds of hours researching the latest findings on this disease and all the factors that can contribute to its amelioration. This research has included discussions with endocrinologists and others in the health field.

Here is a list of some well-known diabetics who have helped to shape the world despite their handicap. What others have done, you can do also. Several books have such a list, but the one by Dr. A. Rubin is the best I have seen. Here is a summary:

List of Celebrities with Diabetes Mellitus

Miss World
Nicole Johnson

Actors
Jackie Gleason
Jack Benny
James Cagney
Spencer Tracy
Halle Berry

Actresses
Mary Tyler Moore
Elizabeth Taylor
Mae West

Artists
Walt Kelly (the Pogo comic strip)
Paul Cézanne

Authors
Mario Puzo (author of *The Godfather)*
Ernest Hemingway
H. G. Wells

Singers and Musicians
Jerry Garcia (The Grateful Dead)
Johnny Cash
Carol Channing (Hello Dolly)
Dizzy Gillespie
Mahalia Jackson
Elvis Presley
Kate Smith

Composer
Giacomo Puccini

Athletes
Arthur Ashe
Jackie Robinson
Catfish Hunter
Ty Cobb
Billie Jean King

Business
Ray Kroc (founder of the McDonald's chain)

Politicians
Gamel Abdel-Nasser
Yuri Andropov
Nikita Kruschev
Mikhail Gorbechev
Menachem Begin
King Fahd
Clinton Anderson
Fiorello La Guardia

Josip Tito
Winnie Mandela, by association
President Clinton's mother, by association

Inventor
Thomas Alva Edison

Dr. Rubin suggests that the personal strengths developed by many famous diabetics also helped them to fame in their professional calling. "Or maybe their diabetes forced them to be stronger, more perseverant, and therefore more successful."

"The...last few blocks to complete freedom of choice for those with diabetes will come down as you show that you can safely do anything that a person without diabetes can do."

—Alan L. Rubin, M.D., *Diabetes for Dummies*, pp. 10-11.

Even more encouraging are these words: "If God be for us, who [or what] can be against us?" (Rom 8:31).

1

Diabetes—The Mystery Disease

The chief topic of this book is adult onset or type 2 diabetes, since over 93 percent of diabetics belong in this category. Practically every technical work on adult-onset diabetes stresses how much information remains to be understood regarding it. Most researchers prefer to think of it as a syndrome, a collection of diseases rather than just one. All admit that its cause is unknown, though we know it can have up to 50 genetic sources triggered by a variety of factors. These include other hormonal irregularities, drugs, stress, but chiefly obesity, consumption of junk foods, and sedentary life-style. In contrast, type 1 diabetes is often the result of a viral infection or an allergic reaction to early milk consumption.

While over 90 percent of diabetics appear to fit a well-known pattern, the rest are challenging exceptions. More and more endocrinologists talk about "bioindividuality," which means that each of us differs in our reactions to drugs, exercise, food and drink, etc. And even more important is the fact that we all inherited different genetic defects.

An interesting example is the landmark study, the DCCT (the Diabetes Control and Complications Trial), the results of which were announced at Reno in 1993. While only involving type 1 diabetics, the key concluding word of CONTROL has been universally regarded as applying to both type 1 and type 2 diabetics. Commenting on the results of the study, Drs. Diana and Richard Guthrie state:

> …We need to obtain and maintain a high degree of control in order to prevent complications of diabetes. This has resulted in a great impetus to develop new methods of management. Various people are searching for new ways to provide this management using various kinds of protocols, algorithms, and mathematical formulas. It's been shown that the exchange system does not fit well into this kind of management, so new diet regimens or

methodologies are being searched for and researched in order to improve control.

—Diana W. Guthrie, R.N., Ph.D., and Richard A. Guthrie M.D.,
The Diabetes Sourcebook, p. 181.

It is interesting that the authors do not say "blood sugar control," but just use the latter word only. In this they are completely faithful to those who announced their conclusions from DCCT. Not "blood sugar control" but "control" was the word chosen to convey the researchers' conclusion. Of course, this did include the former, but was not intended to be limited to it because of the vital fact of bioindividuality.

Complications are NOT determined just by elevated blood glucose, but by a group of factors in which glucose is prominent but not always chief. Obesity, nutrition, hypertension,[1] use of tobacco, sedentary life-style, and incipient coronary heart disease (CHD)—all play a significant part in determining whether the patient has complications, and if so, of what sort. For example, young athletic diabetics are rarely troubled with neuropathy, and nonsmokers are not liable to have amputations.

In view of these facts, competent researchers are stressing the need, not just for blood glucose control but for obedience to all the known laws of health. They advocate losing weight for the obese, reducing blood pressure (usually for the same group), learning to manage stress, the need for regular physical activity, and using a carefully selected diet. In therapy itself a variety of treatments may be offered and tried in order to suit individual needs. While most people are better off for getting as close to a vegetarian diet as possible, a small percentage seem to metabolize animal foods better. Many long-time diabetics are unable to exercise vigorously and, for them, the other forms of control become more essential—especially diet.

Because diabetics are many times more likely to die from CHD, most nutritionists recommend a diet in which saturated fat plays only a very minor part. This means that animal products and dairy products should be used sparingly; also such vegetarian products as palm and coconut oils. Sadly, it must be acknowledged that conventional diet therapy for overweight individuals usually has a failure rate of greater than 90 percent. Only those with very high motivation succeed—such as that which exists in the Christian who believes that his or her body is a temple of God.

One paradoxical proof of bioindividuality is the fact that, despite tight glucose control, some will develop serious complications, whereas some who seem careless of control will not. There is no substitute for faith in divine providence accompanying our very best efforts. Without the latter, difficulties may arise within five years or considerably less, causing diabetics to move from diet therapy alone to pill or insulin usage and their many problems and dangers. For those prepared to live a disciplined life, this can often be avoided.

The title of this chapter is of great importance. Only when it is clearly understood how mysterious diabetes is in nature and, therefore, in methods of therapy, can patients be safe, guarded from unnecessary injury to health, and doctors from error. Anyone familiar with the history of diabetic research realizes that we are only now on the fringes of knowledge concerning this disease, which is the fastest-growing organic epidemic in the Western world in this the 21st century. Even the distinction now commonly made between the two major types of diabetes only came into clear focus in the lifetime of many of us. Healing approaches have been somewhat of a pendulum swing, moving from one extreme to another, and the pendulum has not yet ceased to move. The original approach of near starvation had obvious perils.

With the discovery of insulin by Banting and Best, millions of lives were ultimately to be saved, but after some years it became apparent that there was a new peril not originally seen by diabetic therapists. Cardiovascular diseases became the most common cause of death among diabetics on insulin. Now came the emphasis on a diet consisting of approximately 60 percent carbohydrates. That has predominated until the pronouncement this decade by the ADA that dietary therapy must be individualized, and that 60 percent carbohydrate intake should no longer be held as the standard rule. And over the decades the vast majority of diabetics who have had the disease for many years developed life-threatening complications. While endocrinologists are conscientious, diligent, and intelligent, their results are rarely satisfying to themselves or their patients.

Progress in the perception of all truth is like the coming in of the tide, progress on the whole but with ebb and flow. It was a great advance to learn after many years that diabetes was not just one disease. Discovery of insulin was a tremendous peak in diabetic therapy. The need to counsel diabetics against the overconsumption of cholesterol-laden foods was another advance, though it has some intelligent critics. Dr. Isadore Rosenfeld offers wise counsel:

> The treatment of diabetes remains a subject of great controversy. This is important for you to appreciate, since the second opinion about any problem in diabetes may differ totally from the first, not necessarily on the merits

of the case, but because the physicians involved happen to subscribe to opposite schools of thought.

...If you are middle-aged, are found to be diabetic, and are given insulin despite the fact that you have no symptoms, ask for a second opinion, from a diabetologist.

Some years ago, the observations were made that certain oral medications, chemically related to the sulfa drugs, could reduce blood sugar levels. These agents were not nearly effective enough to substitute for insulin in a young diabetic, but they were initially prescribed for almost everybody else with high blood sugar...

The oral medication seemed to result in a greater number of deaths from heart disease than did the treatments consisting of insulin or diet alone...At least one of these medications has been withdrawn from the market in the United States, and others now carry a label stating that their use may be hazardous to your health.

—*Second Opinion,* p. 60-62.

Eugene D. Robin, formerly of the faculties of Harvard Medical School and the University of Pittsburgh Medical School and Stanford University School of Medicine, has lectured to medical groups all over USA. He has written a book entitled *Matters of Life and Death.* This book has to do with the risks verses the benefits of medical care. On page 74, Dr. Robin says:

Biguanidines, an oral drug used to treat diabetes, produced a life-threatening and sometimes fatal complication, acidosis, a condition in which the blood becomes highly acidic, as a result of which the patient may die.

Every profession has its own hazards. The great temptation for physicians is the compulsion to do something for patients—even when that "something" may leave the patient worse off then before. At times there can be a distinct difference between the goals of curing disease and caring for the sufferer. It is possible for the former goal to interfere with the latter. On one occasion, decades ago, when for some months I was suffering from a functional disorder, I was sent from specialist to specialist without any good result. Then one of the finest physicians I have ever met quizzed me very closely about my daily program and urged me to drastically reduce a numbers of things I felt called to accomplish. I did so, and the problem disappeared. Sir William Osler, pioneer of Canadian medicine, once said: "one of the first duties of the physician is to educate the masses not to take medicine."

But what is the conscientious practitioner to do? Confronted by someone with a real problem, he or she must act on their behalf. At this stage most endocrinologists fall back upon accepted medical procedures regardless of his or her own doubts. To do otherwise is to risk suspension from the medical profession. How, then, can change and improvement ever take place? Only when some take the risk of forsaking unproven medical therapeutic traditions.

On the other side of the equation is the poor human nature of typical patients. They are in no mood to be told to jump a horizontal pole that is clearly too high for them. From their very first months as interns, physicians learn the reluctance of most human beings to change their habits and practices. Patients come to a physician not primarily for advice on life-style but for a quick remedy for existing symptoms. It is not so much advice that many of them seek, but a pill or an injection. Because of this sorry condition of human nature, some young physicians leave medicine.

What does all this mean for the diabetic? Aware that the cause and cure of diabetes are shrouded in mystery, the diabetic must find a physician believed to be open-minded, well read, and more concerned about the well-being of the patient than his or her own ease. The responsibility of the patient, however, does not end there. While it would not be possible for patients to master the professional jargon found in the textbooks, they can read widely enough to find out the current issues and perhaps discover what is the true cutting edge of therapy.

Millions of type 2 diabetics around the world are given oral medication every year. There is no doubt that this has its legitimate place, but there have been more and more warnings that they are too frequently prescribed and too carelessly to the great harm of multitudes. The evidence for this is found in one of the most recent textbooks on diabetes entitled *Clinical Diabetes Mellitus*, edited by John K. Davidson. I have quoted from it in chapter 10.

For the Christian, there is the comfort of knowing that there are no mysteries with God. He alone understands all problems, all situations, and all people and knows what is best for each one of us. His providence has been at work in the world of medicine to the blessing of untold millions, but he has never given his own prerogative of infallibility to any group of men or women on this planet. Therefore, make inquiries regarding an endocrinologist who is successfully helping diabetics, and enroll yourself under his or her care. But do not be afraid to ask questions, and read as much of the current literature on the topic as you can.

Then carefully and prayerfully reason both from the known facts and from cause to effect in actual experimentation.

Note the experience of Dr. Diana Schwarzbein who now runs the endocrinology institute of Santa Barbara. For a time Dr. Schwarzbein worked at a famous clinic in California that had once been the premier diabetes center in the United States. All her new patients were type 2 diabetics, and she found they did not improve. She says:

> I had seen too many diabetics have legs amputated, too many who required kidney dialysis or who had scars down the middle of their chests from coronary bypass grafting. Working with diabetics meant that I would have to watch people inevitably get sicker and die.
>
> …Because the patients were all new to me, I spent a full hour with each one, obtaining a detailed history. I will never forget the anxiety I felt when they would begin by saying, "I hope you won't tell me the same thing all the other doctors have said. It just doesn't work for me." They complained of higher blood-sugar levels and higher blood pressure, despite medication, and of chronic fatigue, weight gain, and abnormal cholesterol profiles.

> —*The Schwarzbein Principle*, pp. xv-xvi.

Dr. Schwarzbein said that all her newly diagnosed diabetics were put on the American Diabetes Association diet—a low-calorie, high-carbohydrate, low-fat, low-protein program. Those on insulin gained weight and, with the added weight, came increased blood pressure. Then many were given drugs to lower the blood pressure with the result in some cases that their blood sugars became worse. It was a vicious cycle. After following the "standard diabetes care," they felt awful. Dr. Schwarzbein concluded that the typical therapy failed to help large numbers of patients, and she saw the high carbohydrate consumption as a major reason for the failure. I do not see light in all the dietetic approaches of Dr. Schwarzbein but, in this particular area, I believe she is "spot on."

In case you think I am too skeptical, two points should be made. The first is, we should thank God with all our hearts for the wonders of modern medicine. But second, remembering how the best of men and women are prone to error, we should never cease to demand evidence for the medical positions doctors take. There have been multitudes of instances where failure in this regard has brought untold harm to huge numbers of people. Dr. Eugene Robin listed many of these to over a hundred medical audiences before writing his book *Matters of Life and*

Death. Some of the damaging medical practices Dr. Robin listed included the following:

- Diethylstilbestrol (DES) to prevent spontaneous abortion.

- High oxygen exposure and blindness in children. (Many premature infants were treated with high oxygen concentrations and by the 1950's the disease thus caused was the leading cause of blindness in children.)

- Internal mammary artery ligation for coronary artery disease. (A chest artery was surgically tied to increase blood supply to the heart but the surgery proved to be valueless.) Huge numbers of patients experienced this surgical procedure and suffered pain, disability, and occasionally death by way of result.

- Ileal bypass and obesity. This again was a surgical procedure and it was designed to enable patients to lose weight but in actual result it caused liver disease, arthritis and even death. It is no longer practiced.

- Tonsillectomy in children. Millions of children suffered this surgery on almost a routine basis and in most cases the operation was without justification. We now know that the excision of tonsils handicaps the body's immune system. Which is not to deny that in very rare cases it is justified. We should not forget that despite overwhelming evidence that indicates no general benefit it remained the single most common procedure in children, approximately 400,000 being performed annually in the United States.

- Thyroid removal or thyroid suppression by drugs as treatment for coronary artery disease or chronic lung disease. The result? A further burden of hypothyroidism.

- Leukemia-causing agents for trivial or inappropriate diseases. Potent drugs wrongly used led to the late development of leukemia.

- Thalidomide. This story is well known. Millions of women early in pregnancy were assigned this drug causing an epidemic of children born severely deformed. Approximately 8,000 cases in West Germany alone testified to the error of this therapy.

- Radiation for acne. Resulting often in cancer of the skin.

- Entero-Vioform and neurologic disease. This drug was prescribed for millions of Japanese patients who had mild intestinal problems and resulted in more than 10,000 deaths.

Dr. Robin, of course, listed other man-made epidemics and then declared that he offered only a partial listing. See pages 74-77 of his book published in the 1980's by the Stanford Alumni Association. The book has also appeared under another title: *Medical Care can be Dangerous to Your Health.*

Yes, diabetes is, indeed, a mysterious disease. I suspect that in the West the main proportion of sufferers are overweight, sedentary, and consuming a refined diet. But not everybody who is overweight, sedentary, and not eating "food as grown" is diabetic. All experts acknowledge that the cause of diabetes is unknown. The disease is furthermore a mystery as to cure. The possibility of cure is usually denied, though Nathan Pritikin claims to have helped hundreds of diabetic sufferers to return to normal living, no longer suffering the symptoms of this disease. His successes were universally in the category just mentioned—the overweight, the underexercised, and the consumers of junk food. He claimed no success from sufferers of type 1 diabetes, and there were many others among type 2 patients that he was unable to help in any permanent way.

Should we be discouraged? Not at all! Practical affairs of life are governed by a weight of evidence, never by demonstration. On the way that leads to the city of God there is no difficulty the Christian faces for which God is not made provision, not a sorrow for which heaven has no healing balm, not an infirmity that our Maker and Redeemer is unable to strengthen.

Footnotes

1. Approximately fifteen percent of people with diabetes with hypertension have a blood pressure as low as 140/90, and only 5 percent have a blood pressure down to 130/85. Thirty-five years ago doctors did not regard high blood pressure as particularly serious, but we know much better today when approximately one in every five Americans suffers from this complaint which triggers so many others. Dr. Gerald Reaven of Stanford, a leading researcher, believes that scientific studies establish that 60 percent of hypertension cases are caused by hyperinsulinism. Far better than the therapy of diuretics and beta-blockers is the primary treatment of exercise and nutritional changes. Just losing weight can often return blood pressure to normal. The risk for high blood pressure in obese American adults is nearly six times that of the nonobese of the same age and sex groups. While the initial concern of specialists with diabetics is their blood glucose numbers, in many cases hypertension plays a larger role in bringing on CHD and pre-

cipitating stroke or kidney problems. We quote from the textbook *Clinical Diabetes Mellitus*:

> A strong association between diabetes, hypertension, obesity and atherosclerosis has been known for more than 75 years. Today, it is established that both the incidence and prevalence of systolic and diastolic hypertension occur with an increased frequency in diabetic patients.

—p. 663.

The Framingham study, which included 239 adults with diabetes, showed that the average blood pressure was more than 6mm/Hg higher in diabetic men and over twelve mm/Hg in diabetic women. It is usual to find a higher systolic blood pressure in borderline diabetics newly diagnosed. The majority of patients with diabetic nephropathy have hypertension. It is important to understand that hypertension often proceeds the diagnosis of NIDDM, showing that it is not the blood glucose as such that is the cause of hypertension.

2

Why Me?

When I was in my seventieth year, I received the diagnosis of diabetes from my physician. I rejected it. It was clearly another case of medical error. After all, one in every seven tests yields a wrong result. This was one of those, or so I thought.

I had been a vegetarian for more than half a century and a vegan for many years. Every day I exercised from one to three hours, studying, praying, or planning as I did so. For half a century, my life had been crammed with activity, but there had been no sickness except the flu. About forty times around the globe was my air mileage on itineraries for gospel seminars. Had I not also lectured on health and preventive medicine for ten years over television (channel 42, northern California) and written a popular book on the topic, *Worth More Than a Million*, which had circulated by the thousands, particularly to viewers?

But I was wrong. I did have diabetes. I knew most diabetics were overweight, inactive, and lived on junk food. None of that fitted me. Ultimately, I accepted the verdict after a hemoglobin A1c blood test (a test which shows the average of the blood sugars over the previous 2-3 months).

A specialist said I had low levels of leptin but was extremely sensitive to its effects. He felt that this could be responsible for my diabetes, and that it was probably genetic. Leptin is a hormone produced in fat. It was discovered in the OB knockout gene mouse in 1994. Leptin sends a message to the brain via the central nervous system that there is enough energy stored in fat for use, and it acts as an off-switch for the appetite. Leptin interacts with insulin. Apparently diabetes could have overtaken me in my forties, and I was fortunate to have arrived at seventy without it. But I remembered that I had experienced diabetic symptoms (gum disease, more frequent urination, dizziness) since I had a traumatic accident in Russia some six years previously. I was preaching in a village hall, passed out and had a bad fall from the platform. I suffered a concussion and many bruises. I also tore the meniscus in my knee, and that took 4-5 years to mend.

It is a normal reaction to initially reject bad news. When, however, we yield to the weight of evidence, we then ask "Why me?"

Of course, a ready response could be "Why not you?" Do you remember the story at the beginning of Luke 13?

> Now there were some present at that time who told Jesus about the Galileans whose blood Pilate had mixed with their sacrifices. Jesus answered, "Do you think that these Galileans were worse sinners than all the other Galileans because they suffered this way? I tell you, no! But unless you repent, you too will all perish. Or those eighteen who died when the tower in Siloam fell on them—do you think they were more guilty than all the others living in Jerusalem? I tell you, no! But unless you repent, you too will all perish."

They had, by implication, asked Jesus the wrong question. A more appropriate one would have been this. "How is it that God hasn't taken away my life since I got out of bed this morning?" All of us are sinners. We have all committed the greatest sins it is possible to commit. We have broken the two great commandments—not once or twice but always. None of us has loved God with all our being, or our neighbor as ourselves.

But we are believers. Why us? John Newton who wrote "Amazing Grace" and other wonderful hymns had an answer of sorts. He said: "No unbeliever has a right to complain about anything; and no believer has a reason to complain about anything."

Those of us who believe that God attends the funeral of every sparrow, and counts the hairs of our heads, must not think and act as though God falls asleep or is in absentia. If chance is on the throne, God is not, and vice versa. To Pilate, Christ said: "Thou couldest have no power at all against me unless it were given thee from above" (John 19:11). Every child of God must give the same answer regarding each tragedy, frustration, disappointment, and loss.

Joseph told his brethren regarding their wicked course of action, "Ye meant it for evil, but God intended it for good." King David's reply to a hot-headed soldier bent on slaying one who had maligned the monarch was, "God has bidden him, 'Curse David'" (2 Sam 16:11). The psalmist knew this secret and therefore wrote: "My times are in thy hand" (Psa 31:15). And the Old Testament chronicler urged upon complainers a real mouth stopper: "This thing is from me" (1 Kings 12:24). If we truly believe that all things work together for good, and that nothing can separate us from the love of God in Christ, we shall be prepared to drink the cup of shock and pain. Give thanks it is not an ocean. Give thanks one can still walk and talk and live and love. Indeed, diabetics can do anything other people can do, except eat carbohydrates with impunity.

Paul, the man whom God used more than any other man who ever lived, except our Lord, was always immersed in trouble up to his eyebrows. Few lives could match his for stress and strain. He wrote something that we all need to learn.

> And lest I should be exalted above measure through the abundance of the revelation, there was given to me a thorn in the flesh, the messenger of Satan to buffet me, lest I should be exalted above measure. For this thing I besought the Lord thrice, that it might depart from me. And he said unto me, **my grace is sufficient for thee: for my strength is made perfect in weakness.** Most gladly therefore will I rather glory in my infirmities, that the power of Christ may rest upon me. Therefore I take pleasure in infirmities, in reproaches, in necessities, in persecutions, in distresses for Christ's sake: for when I am weak, then am I strong.

> —2 Cor 12:7-10 KJV.

Scripture says there is "all joy and peace in believing." (See Romans 15:13.) The same verse says it is our privilege to "abound in hope." He that spared not his own Son but delivered him up for us all, how shall he not with him also freely give us all things?" (Rom 8:32). That means all things best for us, not all things our cowardly nature might ask.

The diabetic must learn to often repeat the promises of Scripture. Any one of them is worth more than a king's ransom. Try this one often: "If God be for us, who can be against us?" (Rom 8:31), and the one referred to above: "My grace is sufficient for thee." Have you heard Charles Spurgeon's comment on these words? Here it is:

> I have often read in Scripture of the holy laughter of Abraham, when he fell upon his face and laughed; but I do not know that I ever experienced that laughter till a few evenings ago, when this text came home to me with such sacred power as literally to cause me to laugh. I had been looking at its original meaning, and trying to fathom it, till at last I got hold of it this way. 'My grace,' says Jesus, 'is sufficient for thee,' and it looked almost as if it were meant to ridicule my unbelief: for surely the grace of such a one as my Lord Jesus is indeed sufficient for so insignificant a being as I am. It seemed to me as if some tiny fish, being very thirsty, was troubled with fear of drinking the

river dry, and Father Thames said to him, 'Poor little fish, my stream is sufficient for thee.' I should think it is, and inconceivably more.

My Lord seems to say to me, 'Poor little creature that thou are, remember what grace there is in me, and believe that it is all thine. Surely it is sufficient for thee.' I replied, 'Ah, my Lord, it is indeed.' Put one mouse down in all the granaries of Egypt when they were fullest after seven years of plenty, and imagine that one mouse complaining that it might die of famine. 'Cheer up,' says Pharaoh, 'poor mouse, my granaries are sufficient for thee.' Imagine a man standing on a mountain, and saying, 'I breathe so many cubic feet of air in a year; I am afraid that I shall ultimately inhale all the oxygen which surrounds the globe.' Surely the earth on which the man would stand might reply, 'My atmosphere is sufficient for thee.' I should think it is; let him fill his lungs as full as ever he can, he will never breathe all the oxygen, nor will the fish drink up all the river, nor the mouse eat up all the stores in the granaries of Egypt.

Does it not make unbelief seem altogether ridiculous, so that you laugh it out of the house, and say, 'Never come this way any more, for with such a mediatorial fullness to go to, with such a Redeemer to rest in, how dare I for a moment think that my wants cannot be supplied.'

Our great Lord feeds all the fish of the sea, and the birds of the air, and the cattle on the hills, and guides the stars, and upholds all things by the power of his hand, how then can we be straitened for supplies, or be destitute of help? If our needs were a thousand times larger than they are they would not approach the vastness of his power to provide. The Father hath committed all things into his hand. Doubt him no more. Listen, and let him speak to thee: '*My* grace is sufficient for thee. What if thou hast little grace, yet *I* have much: it is my grace thou hast to look to, not thine own, and *my* grace will surely be sufficient for thee.'

John Bunyan has the following passage, which exactly expresses what I myself have experienced. He says that he was full of sadness and terror, but suddenly these words broke in upon him with great power, and three times together the words sounded in his ears, 'My grace is sufficient for thee; my grace is sufficient for thee; my grace is sufficient for thee.' And 'Oh! methought,' says he, 'that every word was a mighty word unto me; as '*My*,' and '*grace*,' and '*sufficient*,' and '*for thee*'; they were then, and sometimes are still, far bigger than others be." He who knows, like the bee, how to suck honey from flowers, may well linger over each one of these words and drink in unutterable content.

—C.H. Spurgeon, *Metropolitan Tabernacle Pulpit*, Vol. XXII, pp.197-198.

There is stress, added stress, in the life of every diabetic. But God has made provision for that also. (See our Appendix C.) Here is a promise for the very worst of days. "I will fear no evil, for thou art with me" (Psa 23). The Christian knows that his sun will rise, that the moon will be full again, that winter gives way to spring, that the cross makes sure the coming, and he or she can cry with Luther: "Lord, do what you will, now that my sins are forgiven."

"For God has not given us the spirit of fear but of power, and love, and a sound mind" (2 Tim 1:7).

3

Carbohydrates—The Heart of the Problem

Here is the paradox of current therapy for diabetics. It is admitted that it is primarily the consumption of carbohydrates that raises blood glucose, yet diabetics are counseled to have a diet consisting chiefly of the very class of foods which causes their trouble. In almost all books on the topic, authors recommend 50-60 percent of calories as carbohydrate. No wonder thousands of type 2 sufferers endure frustration three or more times a day as they endeavor to follow such impossible directions. I am, of course, referring chiefly to those diabetics not taking pills and insulin.

In case anybody should doubt our first premise, I illustrate here typical acknowledgements of the part played by carbohydrates in the raising of blood glucose:

> Note that a person who does not have diabetes will have very little change in blood sugar even after eating a whole box of candy, but the person with diabetes will have an elevated blood sugar.

> —Diana W. Guthrie, R.N., Ph.D., and Richard A. Guthrie, M.D.,
> *The Diabetes Sourcebook*, p. 21.

The foods you eat (primarily the starches or carbohydrates) raise your blood sugar to higher-than-normal levels.

> —*Ibid.*, p.1.

We will concentrate on the well-documented fact involved in carbohydrate ingestion and its effect on blood sugar levels.

—Dr. Rachael F. Heller, *The Carbohydrate Addicts Healthy Heart Program*, p. 88.

Diabetes mellitus, disorder of carbohydrate metabolism resulting from an insufficiency in the production or utilization—or both—of insulin.

—*Encyclopaedia Britannica*, Micropaedia, III:515 (15th edition).

Despite this universally acknowledged fact, that it is carbohydrates that raise blood sugar, the majority of endocrinologists have advocated a high-carbohydrate diet. Why is this so?

Prior to the discovery of insulin in 1921, the usual treatment of diabetes was a semi-fasting state with carbohydrates prohibited.

Dr. Rosenfeld describes the situation as follows:

Leafing through a medical book published in the early 1900s, I found the *symptoms* of diabetes—thirst, frequent urination, weight loss, increased appetite, itching, and coma—accurately described. But although high blood sugar was recognized as the cause, insulin was not destined to be discovered until the 1920s. In this same text, the author stated that most children live only six months to four years after the diagnosis was made. Death in those days came in the form of "exhaustion" or coma. Treatment consisted of an absolute rigid diet without even a trace of sugar or starch…"

—*The Best Treatment*, p. 87.

When carbohydrates were forbidden, diabetics automatically turned to the consumption of large quantities of animal products, which are free of carbohydrates. And the results were disastrous. Even today, heart disease is the main cause of death among diabetics, but early deaths now are considerably less than in the days prior to 1922, when insulin therapy began. As might be expected, a pendulum phenomenon took place. After some decades, patients were shifted from a meat-centered diet to one of carbohydrates. Because diet alone was the treatment for only a minority of sufferers, sulfonylureas (pills) and insulin were used to deal with the carbohydrate consumption.

Treatment by diet alone is the approach recommended in theory by most specialists. Though a minority, millions of people are being treated this way. The more conscientious these people are in endeavoring to keep their blood sugars down, the more frustrated they become because a high-carbohydrate diet won't work for diabetics.

Without medication, it is impossible to keep blood sugars down on a diet that is largely carbohydrate—absolutely impossible.

Estimates of the measurements of glucose in the blood by using urine tests were never very satisfactory, and blood glucose monitors only became available in the mid-eighties. Because of these factors, there was a delay in perceiving the damage that high carbohydrate intake was doing to those type 2 diabetics who were depending on diet alone for blood sugar control. Similarly, it didn't help other diabetic sufferers who, though using insulin and pills, still needed to be disciplined in their eating habits.

In the last thirty years or so, protests have been multiplying. The most vocal has come from Dr. Richard K. Bernstein who was initially treated for diabetes in the 1940s—a time he describes as the Dark Ages of diabetic therapy. He, as a type 1 diabetic, used insulin constantly but found himself developing the disease complications one by one until he almost despaired. After finding a meter designed to distinguish between diabetics in a coma and collapsed alcoholics, Dr. Bernstein began to experiment on himself. It was like the rising of the sun after the darkness of night when he found the connection between his traditional eating habits and elevated blood sugars.

Immediately he began to restrict his carbohydrate consumption with astonishing and gratifying results. In his forties, this engineer decided to become a physician. Not long after his graduation, he set up his own clinic for diabetics with amazing success.

Dr. Bernstein uses animal products freely, an abundance of leafy vegetables, and exercises vigorously every day. Today, many endocrinologists are sympathetic with the protest of Dr. Bernstein, but choose a different therapy—with reduced carbohydrates and a lesser emphasis on animal products. Dr. Alan Rubin is representative of these. Note his words:

> If there were a more controversial area in nutrition for the diabetic person than carbohydrates, I would like to know about it. For years, the American Diabetes Association told people with diabetes that they should be eating 55

to 60 percent of their calories as carbohydrate. Other experts said that that amount was too much. Some even said that that amount was too little. The ADA has now modified its recommendation so that it says in the Clinical Practice Recommendations for 1998: "The percent of carbohydrate will vary and is individualized, based on the individual's eating habits and glucose and lipid (fat) goals." In this section, I give you my suggestions for carbohydrate in your diet based on my reading of the medical literature and my clinical experience. You are free to disagree with me and use whatever level of carbohydrate you like as long as it helps to promote lower blood glucose without increasing blood fats or weight…

Because carbohydrate is the food that raises the blood glucose, which is responsible for the complications of diabetes, it seems right to recommend a diet that is lower in carbohydrate than previously suggested. Furthermore, a major source of coronary artery disease in diabetes is the insulin resistance syndrome (see Chapter 5). Because increased carbohydrate triggers increased triglycerides, which is the beginning of a number of abnormalities that lead to increased coronary artery disease, recommending less carbohydrate on this basis as well seems prudent.

My experience has been that a diet of 40 percent carbohydrate makes controlling my patient's blood glucose much easier.

—Diabetes for Dummies, pp. 125-126.

Many endocrinologists follow the same approach as Rubin and, increasingly, books on diabetes sound a warning against high-carbohydrate diets, or at least allow for the alternative approach. For examples, see our Appendix B.

Almost all modern works on diabetes discuss the Glycemic Index, which categorizes carbohydrate foods according to the rapidity of their digestion and absorption. Dr. David Jenkins, professor of nutrition at the University of Toronto, Canada, pioneered the concept. His purpose was to help people with diabetes, and he has succeeded wonderfully well. Only foods low on the index are recommended, which wipes out the vast majority of popular foods, especially refined products and simple sugars.

However, Dr. Richard Bernstein and many specialists say that people consuming large amounts of food, low on the glycemic index, are still in danger. Only the very lowest on the scale can be recommended. These include soya beans, nuts, and nonstarchy vegetables.

When a diet high in carbohydrates and one high in animal fats and proteins both cause problems, there doesn't seem much left to eat. It creates a huge dilemma for the hungry diabetic intent on treatment by diet alone. I learned about these problems because, on initial diagnosis, I took my blood sugar many times a day. I took it at different times of the day, at different lengths of time after eating. I experimented with foods, both with amount and type. I experimented with exercise. I found that I needed to wait after eating before I exercised. If I didn't, my blood sugar would go up later when I returned from exercise because the food was only partially digested. The glycemic index was a helpful tool, but I found Dr. Bernstein was right that even that could be misleading.

The next chapter describes what I found out, and how it went against what many of the traditional books were giving as the ideal diabetic diet (but not current research).

4

Monounsaturates—Solving the Diabetic's Dietary Dilemma

What I found out from experimentation was that I could eat reasonable amounts of foods with generous amounts of monounsaturates in them and foods very low on the glycemic index, such as soya beans and salad vegetables. This idea, not original with me, but not widely stressed yet, is the most recent arrival in diabetic theory. It is a primary reason for this book, this stress on monounsaturates such as predominate in nuts, avocados, flaxseed, olives, etc. Manuals are appearing suggesting that 45 percent of the diet should consist of these as a healthy alternative to animal products and foods chiefly carbohydrate in nature. Instead of raising cholesterol and tryglicerides, the monounsaturates lower both. The importance of this new approach cannot be overestimated.

Note carefully that I am recommending the whole foods containing monounsaturates, not refined oils. **All refined products are deleterious.**

Nuts are a neglected food, though they are a powerhouse of energy and are rich in vitamins and minerals. The wide range of nuts offers a delicious alternative for those struggling with elevated blood sugars. Eaten with an abundance of leafy vegetables, soya beans, with flavoring can be both enjoyable and safe. Such a diet does not raise the blood glucose to unacceptable levels, and I and others can testify to the benefit of this discovery. The whole beans are better than most soya bean products—with the possible exception of low-carbohydrate soya milk.

I encourage you to experiment yourself. Reason from cause to effect. Remember that no one is identical in his or her reactions to foods or programs, such as exercise. But this chapter summarizes where modern research is heading and will help most of those who apply it.

The *Encyclopedia Britannica* in its article on diabetes has words that should stand out like diamonds. Here they are:

Most individuals with adult-onset diabetes are overfed, underactive, and overweight. Significant alteration on one, two, or all three of these variables can eradicate laboratory evidence of diabetes.

—Volume VI: 837 (15th edition).

Do not pass by the word "most," but esteem it highly. For some diabetics there is no way of eradicating the laboratory evidence of diabetes. But for many it can be done. But how? For a considerable number, just losing weight significantly will do. But what should be said to the majority that cannot be helped so simply?

A diet rich in monounsaturates, low in carbohydrates, accompanied by daily exercise such as thirty to sixty minutes of walking, swimming, cycling, or jogging is the best program for most diabetics.

This means emphasis in the diet plan upon the following vegetables: artichoke, asparagus, beans (green, wax, Italian), bean sprouts, cabbage, carrots, cauliflower, eggplant, greens (collard, mustard), kohlrabi, okra, onions, pea pods (not peas themselves), green peppers, rutabaga, sauerkraut, summer squash, turnips, water chestnuts, and zucchini.

At the same meal, for high-energy resources, nuts should be eaten—chewed very slowly to ensure digestion. Unsalted raw nuts, particularly almonds are the ones to use, but including peanuts, pecans, brazils, hazelnuts, pistachios, walnuts, and, to a lesser extent, cashews (because they are higher in carbohydrate than most nuts). Soya beans, because of their high protein and fat content, slow down the digestion of their carbohydrate and can be used abundantly, including roasted soy nuts.

"But," you may protest, "soyas are the least palatable of all beans." True, but they can be made palatable by adding tahini or nut butters. They and most vegetables become delicious if salsa is added. The peppers in salsa help prevent neuropathy. For salsa, choose those brands that list tomatoes first rather than tomato paste.

"And what do I do for sweetening?" The herbal sweetener, Stevia, is one answer. Stevia (pronounced STEE-vee-uh) comes from a shrub in South America. The inhabitants of Brazil and Paraguay have used its leaves for centuries to sweeten certain of their foods and beverages, and the Japanese have used it since the early 1970s in manufacturing pickles and other products. There has been no evidence over the centuries of any harm in Stevia use. The FDA, as yet, has not licensed it to be sold as a sweetening agent, though they permit its sale as a food additive. Huge amounts ingested at one time MAY have deleterious effects, but that is true of salt and many other things we use daily.

Dr. Bernstein holds that plain = full cream yogurt (with live cultures) is a reasonable food for diabetics. Though high in carbohydrate, its digestion and absorption is slowed because of the high fat and protein content.

The golden rule in many of these dietary issues is to reason from cause to effect. Everybody's metabolism is different to some degree. Make your own glycemic index. By regular monitoring of your blood sugar two hours after meals it becomes apparent what is acceptable for you and what is not.

I have recommended soya beans rather than soy products (with the exception of soya milk). There is a question in some circles about the long-term use of foods containing significant amounts of processed soya. It may be that the industrial processing of soya beans results in some health problems. Only further studies will decide that issue. Meanwhile, it is probably wise to use such products rarely rather than frequently. Only use soya milk made from the whole soya beans, not from soy isolate. As soon as we try to improve on the way God made food, we run into problems. It is the refining of foods that is responsible for much of the ravages of disease in our day. It is particularly the refining of carbohydrates that is a major factor in the epidemic of diabetes.

Another question arises concerning the use of eggs and cheese. While very few dieticians today would recommend the use of red meats, an increasing number are saying that the earlier prejudices against eggs on the ground of their cholesterol content was not altogether well-founded. This recent position results from the knowledge that it is particularly when cholesterol is taken with saturated fats that there is danger in long-term use. But eggs predominate in unsaturated fats, so studies at Harvard and other centers have advised that a moderate use of eggs is probably risk-free. And Parmesan cheese is practically fat and cholesterol free.

For diabetics, the issue is of some importance for there is no carbohydrate in eggs or cheese. They do not raise blood sugar. However, it should be kept in mind that all foods without fiber (all animal products) are constipating, and should only be used with moderation. Except for Parmesan cheese, they also contain cholesterol, which is harmful in excess, especially for those who are sedentary.

By now, it should be apparent that the dietary rules for diabetics are the same as for all others with the exception that they cannot handle foods that are blatantly carbohydrate. There IS carbohydrate in vegetables, soya beans, nuts etc, but it either does not predominate, or, being so made by nature with fat and protein combined, the result on the blood sugar is lessened.

Because, today, three out of every four people in the West die of heart disease or cancer, and because these diseases are chiefly the result of poor nutrition, wisdom in eating pays tremendous dividends. Remember that the whole of dietetics as now understood can be comprehended in principle in a single sentence: "eat fresh, whole foods, chiefly of vegetable origin."

The majority of diabetics have high blood pressure, but a good diet and exercise program can often help remedy or prevent that problem. Many individuals testify that their health is now much better than it was before, since discovering they had diabetes and learning how to treat it.

5

Numbers—Important, but
Not All Important

The conscientious diabetic wishes to keep his or her blood sugar within appropriate bounds and eagerly asks what they may be. The answers over the years differed but not wildly so. In the last decade the conviction has grown that tight control of glucose levels has significant influence on whether and which complications may appear—retinopathy, nephropathy, neuropathy, or cardiovascular symptoms. In about one-third of diabetics, there will be no complications.

I have suggested in the title of this chapter that the numbers to be watched are important but not ALL important. What do I mean? Precisely this: there are several other key factors that play at least as important a role as the glucose levels in determining whether complications will overtake you. Hypertension (high blood pressure), obesity, quality of diet, high cholesterol, high triglycerides, whether you smoke or use much alcohol, and whether you are active or inactive, etc.

Dr. Robert Fredericks uses an illustration in his lectures that suggests that blue cars guzzle gas more than red ones. He is pointing out that unless you have all the facts, you can come to ridiculous conclusions. You can "prove" anything. He says, maybe blue cars are made bigger than red cars. Maybe more men buy blue cars and drive faster. He is spoofing the way a lot of medical research is done. You can look at certain factors such as high cholesterol or high blood sugar as "causes" of disease or you can see them as "associated" with disease. There is a huge difference between these stances. In medicine currently, the tendency is to act as though high blood sugars "cause" the side effects of diabetes, such as neuropathy; and that high cholesterol "causes" heart disease. This is not altogether true. They are both markers that are associated with the diseases, not lone factors causing the side effects or the disease by themselves.

Glucose numbers, on their own, may not decide the health issues, though they are indeed significant. As I have mentioned before, the real outcome of the

DCCT research was the counsel of **control**, not **control blood glucose**, though of course the latter was included in the dictum. The experts could not agree at that convention that lowering blood glucose would always fix the problem.

I recommend that you study the general principles of preventive medicine and apply them[1]. Toxic levels of glucose that continue on unabated are harmful. But do not be concerned by occasional elevated glucose levels. Remember your well-being depends on many factors—not just one.

Footnotes

1. The book *Worth More Than a Million* is a distillation of hundreds of book on the topic of preventive medicine. It is available from Desmond Ford Publications, c/o Good News Unlimited, P. O. Box 6687, Auburn, CA 95604-6687, U.S.A. $25.00, includes shipping and handling.

6

Eating for Health and Joy

All textbooks on therapy for diabetes stress that diet is the cornerstone. Whether one is a type 1 or a type 2 diabetic, whether one is on insulin or pills every day, or whether managing by diet alone, care must be exercised regarding the quality and quantity of food and drink consumed. It is not necessary to go hungry from meal to meal, but it is vital to know which foods have the most impact on your blood glucose and which don't. Fats have no impact on your immediate levels, and the impact of protein is slow and gradual.

To consume pure carbohydrate food or drink is to invite a meteoric rise in glucose levels. The same food or drink eaten at a meal with fat and protein will still register its presence in the blood but at a slower rate. No diabetic should be swallowing large amounts of sugar-laden refreshment between meals.

Even lean meats add to your cholesterol levels. Ideally fat and protein should come from vegetable or dairy sources. Dairy, of course, also contains cholesterol, but overall is probably not as much a threat to health as a heavy meat diet. It is none the less only of secondary value. The nearer one can approach a vegan diet the better.

Now that eggs have been vindicated to some extent by the awareness that their fat is unsaturated, most diabetics can use several each week with safety, preferably from free range or vegetarian fed fowls. Neither egg nor cheese raises glucose levels. Parmesan cheese has neither saturated fat nor cholesterol. You can experiment with buttermilk, to see whether you like it and whether it raises your glucose levels. It has been recommended for diabetics for over a hundred years.

As regards food quantity, the issue revolves around carbohydrate content. Salad greens, such as Romaine lettuce, endive, spinach and parsley contain very little carbohydrate and can be eaten freely. Similarly, vegetables such as cabbage, celery, cucumber, green onion, hot peppers, asparagus, mushroom, and radish contain only small amounts of carbohydrate, and few would overeat on them. Some diabetics, however, will find that anything over one to two cups of these "innocent" foods will elevate their blood sugar numbers. And overcooking these vegetables tends to make them put your blood sugar up. Less rather than more cooking is the rule. Flavorings such as lemon juice, cinnamon, unsweetened pickles, vinegar, basil, chives, oregano, paprika, vanilla, garlic, etc., have negligible amounts of carbohydrate.

The foods that are most satisfying and yet do no harm include nuts of all descriptions, soya beans (but not soya products except soya milk) and vegetables such as eggplant, cauliflower, and broccoli. The individual should experiment with yogurt (full fat and not sweetened) and buttermilk.

The nearer the food is to the way nature provides it, the less likely is that food to raise the blood glucose. Thus raw vegetables are better than cooked, though moderate amounts of cooked vegetables are acceptable. The more finely ground the food, the quicker it raises glucose levels. And the slower a meal is taken with deliberation and pleasure, the slower the blood glucose will rise. There are wheat bran fiber breads such as Bran-a-crisp, which spread with cream cheese are delightful, but too many could be laxative. These are imported from Scandinavia by Inter-Brands Inc., at 3300 N.E. 164th Street, FF3 Ridgefield, WA 98642, U.S.A. The ideal drink, apart from water, is a homemade lemonade from lemons, water and some drops of sweetening Stevia (too much makes it bitter).

The self-control exercised in eating will bring handsome rewards of health and vitality and freedom (for most) from diabetic complications. Remember that, in some respects, you have to be your own doctor. The physician cannot exercise self-discipline on your behalf—it's entirely up to you.

I add two quotations that will help motivate many—one from an old book edited by John H. Knowles, called *Doing Better and Feeling Worse*, and the second, more recent, but bound to become a classic, *A Diabetic Doctor Looks at Diabetes: His and Yours,* by Peter A. Lodewick:

> A program to improve the self-care of patients with diabetes (tertiary prevention) at the University of Southern California resulted in a 50 per cent reduction in emergency-ward visits, a decrease in the number of patients with diabetic coma from 300 to 100 over a two-year period, and the avoidance of 2,300 visits for medications. The theme was, "You must take responsibility for your own health." Savings were estimated at $1.7 million. In other studies involving the care and education of diabetics, hemophiliacs, and other, hospital readmission decreased by over 50 percent. These efforts

resulted in tremendous savings of time and money and reflected vastly improved self-care in cases of chronic disease.

—Doing Better and Feeling Worse, p. 77.

Each person with diabetes has a unique personality, physique, metabolism, and attitude toward diet, exercise, and life in general. Since these factors influence diabetes, the course of the disease will vary with the individual. In some respects, the person with diabetes must be his own doctor, for it is impossible for his physician to understand all the moods, activities and social situations that will affect him. The more the person with diabetes knows about himself, about diabetes, and about the interrelationships of diet, food, exercise, moods and blood sugar, the more he will be able to direct the course of his condition to live many years without complications.

Diet, exercise, insulin, stress, emotion and travel are a few of the factors that affect the control of blood sugar. Since we're all unique, these factors affect each person differently. Even if a physician sees a patient regularly, these effects are difficult to determine. Consequently, the patient needs to evaluate his or her own symptoms and, in a sense, assume the role of being his or her own doctor. Learn as much about diabetes as possible, test blood sugars frequently and learn how to prevent problems of diabetes.

—A Diabetic Doctor Looks at Diabetes—His and Yours, pp. 12, 250-251.

7

Cautions and Counsels for the Practical Control of Diabetes

Remember, nobody knows the cause of diabetes, though we do know many of the triggering factors, including genetics, obesity, poor diet, and a sedentary lifestyle. Most of those items, listed after genetics, apply particularly to type 2 diabetics. A viral attack or allergy to early consumption of cow's milk can trigger type 1 diabetes.

Remember, also, diabetes is called the mysterious disease because, not only do we not know its real cause, but because we cannot cure it, and some of our procedures in therapy are subject to constant correction or revision. The American Diabetic Association has reversed its recommendations more than once, and sensibly so. For example, the admonition of the seventies and eighties to use 50-60 percent of carbohydrates in the diet has been withdrawn, and instead individual needs are emphasized.

The changes in the ADA diet, in a sense, mirror the whole history of diabetic therapy. The original diet for diabetics was one of semi-starvation with practically no carbohydrate. It lacked many essential food elements, and, of course, was deficient in calories. When the trend changed to high-fat diets, largely composed of animal products, the end result was a meteoric rise in heart disease. After the realization in the 1960s of the danger of the consumption of large amounts of animal fats, therapists changed to the advocacy of about 60 percent carbohydrates in the meal plan. The purpose of this was to reduce cardiovascular complications, but it made the control of elevation of blood sugars difficult for anyone trying to avoid medications. Now in the 21st century, there is a swing away from high-carbohydrate levels to the consumption of up to 45 percent of fats, but chiefly monounsaturates. Possibly, the pendulum will cease to swing at this point, for this is the least problematic diet for the diabetic.

With these premises, keep in mind the fact of "bioindividuality." Not everybody responds the same way to triggering factors or therapeutic controls. You must experiment and find what works in your case.

This particularly applies to diet. Very early you must decide whether it is feasible and desirable for you to go the high road of the "diet alone" therapy, or to do what most diabetics ultimately do—depend on pills and insulin.

This decision will influence everything else. For example, you will recall that most diabetic diets are structured to preserve maximum health rather than to keep blood glucose down. As already stated, they include a very high proportion of carbohydrates. For the person depending on diet therapy alone, the typical recommended diet is quite impossible. It will bring disappointment, frustration, rage, and despair.

This book particularly aims at helping those who have chosen the high road of "diet and exercise alone," though it will be helpful for all others as well. I frankly admit that for some, this high road is impossible, and therefore, for such, the high road will be the most life-conserving approach, whatever it is. Some people can't discipline themselves to such a strict diet. Others will have elevated glucose numbers however careful they are about their diet, because of the type of diabetes they have.

For those relying on diet alone to control their diabetes (backed up by abundant and regular physical activity), certain caveats must be added. Here they are:

1. People respond differently to different foods, but in general for almost all not using pills or insulin, even moderate amounts of overt carbohydrates (grains, dairy products, sugars, fruit, most legumes) will push the figure for blood glucose up way beyond what it should be.

2. Don't be discouraged if after your best efforts the figure after two hours is well over 200. Occasional peaks or even weeks of them have little overall significance, but what becomes the average over a long period is vital.

3. It is not the brief peak of high blood glucose that is the primary problem, but its remaining high. Many diabetics experience constant high levels—for most of the time between meals. This is not good. But the occasional high figure up to 250 is not as important, if it does not remain there. If you are physically active, a fast walk can bring it down within about half an hour.

4. Glucose monitors are not infallible. I have more than one and, when surprised by a particular high reading, I take another one immediately with

another machine. Read your manual carefully to see whether you need to add about 12 percent to the figure provided by your monitor to find the actual figure assumed by therapeutic guides. Keep in mind also that even a good monitor can often be out by about 10 percent. Having two different monitors for unusual readings is an aid to peace of mind and a more accurate understanding of the facts. If your meter reads L and won't register, it is because the environment is too cold. Put it in the sun, under your armpit, or near the stove for some minutes, and try again.

5. It is possible that, on occasion, a large preceding meal can accelerate the rise of glucose after the next intake of food.

6. For most diabetics it is the quality of the food, not primarily the quantity, which affects the blood glucose. However, immoderate amounts of even low glycemic foods do have an impact. But it is not nearly as strong as when the wrong quality of food is consumed—i.e., foods that are mainly carbohydrate.

7. All foods contain fat, protein, and carbohydrate and are usually classified according to which of the three predominates. (When we say "all food" we mean those in their natural state—not processed oils or refined grains or sugars.)
    It is imperative to use foods high in fat at the beginning of the meal (viz., avocados, olives, nuts, seeds such as flax or sesame, and, for a change, eggs or cheese or both). Failure to do this at the right time will cause the blood sugar to rise too quickly and too high.

8. For most diabetics relying on diet therapy alone, the following should constitute the bulk of every meal:

    •   Leafy vegetables like lettuce, cabbage and kale and foods like radishes, eggplant, cauliflower, broccoli, mushrooms, cucumbers, peppers, lemons, limes, tomatoes, and an occasional green apple, etc.). Cooked vegetables tend to put the blood sugar up faster.

    •   Polyunsaturated and monounsaturates in general should constitute the bulk of every meal. These include all seeds (e.g., flax, sunflower, and sesame); all kinds of nuts (cashews contain the most carbohydrate and should be used in lower quantities—note that nuts are really a type of seed); plus avocados, soybeans, and olives (preferably olives carefully processed without too much salt)

- Soya beans, in a marvelous way, combine fat, protein, and carbohydrate, but are an extremely low glycemic food and can be eaten freely. They should be initially soaked at least overnight and that water drained off and then cooked very slowly (pressure-cooking may harm the protein content). They are tasteless on their own, so read on. (This endorsement of soya beans does not apply to soy products except soya milk and tofu.)

9. Many diabetics have found that the use of fatty foods at the beginning of the meal slows down the rise in blood sugar. Using some nuts, avocado, olives, eggs, cheese, meat, fish or fowl should constitute the bulk of the first course. We list meat, fish or fowl though we do not think such items are necessary for most people. On the downside, they lack dietary fiber and are subject to disease. But because animal foods are almost devoid of carbohydrate, their use may be considered the lesser of two evils.

10. Salads and soya beans can be made tasty and palatable by the use of salsa and nut butters or tahini. The peppers contain elements that help to ward off neuropathies and are consequently of great importance. So don't be afraid of "hot" salsa—the pepper ingredient is just what diabetics need.

11. An excellent breakfast "cereal" is ground up flax seed and soya milk but choose a soya milk low in carbohydrate. (One must form the habit of reading labels closely. Anything over 12 grams of carbohydrate in a large glass of soya milk is too high. There are brands such as Silk which are lower, especially in the "plain" style. Read on for how to flavor it.)

12. Stevia, though not passed by the FDA as a sweetener, is widely used for that purpose throughout the world and has been so for centuries. It is possible that huge amounts constantly consumed could do damage, but there is no evidence that moderate usage carries any risk. Don't use too much at a time, or the taste is unacceptable. About ten drops to a glass is usually sufficient. Stevia can be purchased at most health-food stores. The liquid form may be better than the powdered, but let each experiment for him or herself.

13. Instead of store-bought biscuits, make your own from a combination of ground seeds (flax, sunflower, sesame, etc.), blended cooked soya beans and soya milk and salt. Spread with nut butter. They can be sweetened with non-caloric sweeteners, included in the mixture before baking. Again, I use Stevia.

14. The reading of labels on food products is essential. Similarly, one should learn from the appropriate books the carbohydrate content of all foods eaten. On average, one gram of carbohydrate raises the blood sugar 3, 4, or 5 points for those who weigh 200 lbs., 150 lbs., and 100 lbs. respectively. The speed with which blood sugar is raised depends on many factors. Very ripe fruit contains more sugar; foods reduced to a mush, such as creamed corn, instead of whole grain raise the levels quickly. Similarly the juice of an orange (instead of the orange itself) and all other juices will raise glucose levels faster. The drier the food and the more it requires chewing, the slower will be the rise in blood sugar.

That is it for the dietary caveats. One more general caution should be given. Never forget that while "control" and "discipline" are key words in diabetic therapy, this term applies to more than just blood sugar levels. It is true that fish and red meats have no carbohydrates, and do not elevate the glucose in the blood. However, it is also true that they contain cholesterol. Too much cholesterol, consumed along with saturated fat, is responsible, in part, for the cardiovascular disease that has always been the chief cause of death for most diabetics.[1]

Therefore, if one chooses to eat meat or fish, it should be in moderate amounts, remembering also that, these days, most animal products are not what they were centuries ago. Chickens are cruelly caged and kept from natural movement. Fish is often tainted with industrial effluent, such as mercury.

Likewise those animals raised for veal. Other livestock also are fed with huge amounts of antibiotics and hormones. Mad cow disease that leads to a variant of Creuzfeld-Jakobs disease may be a shadow of things to come. The nearer one can get to the diet of Eden the better. Nevertheless, one must be content with the best available under the circumstances. An absolute purist could die young.

The life-style, in general, must be under strict discipline—not only your eating habits, but the way you rest and exercise in particular. About one hour after a meal or an hour and a half is the time for vigorous exercise—not before, as it would interrupt digestion. Walking is the best all-around exercise, but the more vigorous it is, the more useful in reducing the blood glucose levels. A fast walk reduces these levels by one to two per minute.

Those who are fit enough to jog will find jogging can reduce glucose numbers by three or more per minute. Remind yourself continually that exercise is an invisible insulin for many diabetics. It is not a cure-all, but after diet it comes the next best. If diet and exercise combined fail to keep your glucose from unacceptably high elevations, medication will be necessary—either pills or insulin. And insulin injections are by far the safer of the two therapies. Insulin cannot be taken by mouth, as it is destroyed in the stomach; but the day may come when it can be administered through adhesive patches. An insulin pump at present costs between $3,000 and $4,000.

Another motivator to regular exercise is the awareness that, if the habit is delayed, the practice may become impossible. About 70 percent of those who have been hospitalized because of diabetic complications are unable to exercise. Many of those complications would have been avoided had exercise been a daily affair (better still—two to three times daily). The heart, kidneys, and eyes are very dependent on the quality of blood circulation. Exercise enhances this in such a way as to either ward off or slow down the development of heart, eye, kidney, and neurological disease.

Not only as regards consumption of animal products is control necessary, but you must shun the use of refined foods, (especially refined oils, cereals, and sugars), and the excessive use of salt. Some diabetics can handle moderate amounts of plain yogurt (with normal not low fat content), buttermilk, and cottage cheese. Experiment, but keep them also to a minimum. Eggs with their unsaturated fat may not be as harmful as long believed, but, if used, should be chosen from free-range fowls and used moderately.

Discipline is a key word for diabetic control, and in one sense its practice is a key to living in general. It applies to all the habits of thought and action. The diabetic who learns to chew deliberately and eat slowly, for example, will reap the dividend of a slower glucose rise. The one who makes it a habit to walk an hour or so after every meal will earn yet even more benefit.

Many will decide to depend on pills or insulin rather than diet alone. They should recall that the sulfonylureas and other pills have been the subject of fierce controversy over recent decades. Insulin is probably safer, though it also has some risks—chiefly that of inducing hypoglycemic attacks.

The average diabetic can spend with ease at least $1,000 a year on elementary aspects of diabetic therapy such as insulin needles, test strips for monitors, and the monitors themselves, as well as the lancets for the monitors. It is widely agreed that insulin needles need not be replaced for each fresh use. A single needle may suffice for the injections of a week. You can change it when it is blunt. Even the lancet can be used many times before replacing.

Sometimes harder to control than any of the above factors is the matter of stress. Adrenaline and cortisol, produced in situations that are dangerous or harassing, raise the blood sugar. A typical public speaker could find his or her levels raised by a hundred after a presentation. This is not of great significance for occasional events, but constitutes a real hazard for those whole lives seem universally stressful.

Bodily movement and deep breathing can reduce the impact of stress and, at another level, the practice of the presence of God.

Learn to say: "I will fear no evil, for Thou art with me," whenever the situation demands it.

Footnotes

1. Hitherto, cholesterol in this book has been treated in a general and simplistic manner. We should now be more specific. While Nathan Pritikin was emphatic that total cholesterol was what mattered, most researchers in the past two decades have not agreed with him. The prevailing wisdom now is that it is the ratio between the total cholesterol figure and the HDL lipoprotein, which is significant. LDLs are the dangerous particles and ideally should not exceed 100, while the HDLs should exceed 45. The lower the ratio between the total figure and the HDL number the better, and it needs remedying if 4.5 or over.

An increasing number of diabetic specialists are insisting that hyperinsulinemia may be more detrimental than a high cholesterol figure. Among these are Doctors Richard K. Bernstein and Calvin Ezrin—both highly respected in their field. These argue that it is a high carbohydrate diet, which causes hyperinsulinemia and elevated triglycerides, subsequently triggering heart disease.

In Dr. Bernstein's most recent work, we read these very significant lines: "The importance of elevated serum insulin levels (hyperinsulinemia) as a cause of heart disease and hypertension has taken on such importance that a special symposium on this subject was held at the end of the 1990 annual meeting of the ADA. A report in the subsequent issue of the journal *Diabetes Care* quite appropriately points out that 'there are few available methods of treating diabetes that do not result in hyperinsulinemia' unless the patient is following a low-carbohydrate diet."—*Dr. Bernstein's Diabetic Solution*, p. 313.

Also worthy of close study is a note found at the foot of page 314 of Dr. Bernstein's Book. Here it is: "If your physician finds all of this hard to believe, he might read the seventy articles and abstracts on this subject contained in the Proceedings of the Fifteenth International Diabetes Foundation Satellite Symposium on "Diabetes and Macrovascular Complications," *Diabetes*, 45, Supplement 3, July, 1996. Also worth reading is "Effects of Varying Carbohydrate Content of Diet in Patients with Non-Insulin Dependant Diabetes Mellitus," by Garg, *et al.*, *Jnl Amer Med Assoc*, 1994; 271:1421-1428.

Dr. Calvin Ezrin says something very similar in *The Type 2 Diabetes Diet Book*. Speaking of insulin he writes: "Until recently the malevolent side of the hormone has been ignored...It is the fat-building hormone generating triglycerides from carbohydrate precursors in the liver and also in adipose tissue where they are stored as energy reserves...Insulin is the second most powerful salt-retaining hormone next to aldosterone. Without excessive intake of calories, it can produce rapid weight gain from fluid retention alone." (page 285).

8

"Cures" That Don't

Having tried at least half a dozen of them, I speak with some conviction. None of the herbs or medications recommended by popular authors as a cure for diabetes has been clinically demonstrated as effective. That's it. That's despite the 700 or so claimants.

Dr. Alan Rubin has an excellent chapter in his *Diabetes for Dummies* on this topic. It is Chapter 17. He's giving three warnings in particular. Here they are in summary:

- *If the treatment has been around for a long time but is not generally used, don't trust it.* A treatment, which has been around a long time and really works, would have been tried in an experimental study where some people take it, and some don't. Doctors' medical texts recommend drugs that pass that test.

- *If it sound too good to be true, it usually is.* An example would be the claims about chromium improving blood glucose levels. The study that "proves" it was done on chromium-deficient people, a situation that does not exist in the United States.

- *Anecdotes are not proof of the value of a treatment or a test.* The favorable experience of one or a few people is not a substitute for a scientific study. If they did seem to respond to the drug, it may be for entirely different reasons.

Chromium is the most touted cure, but no studies on people have demonstrated benefit, despite Dr. Rosenfeld's belief in its value. Chromium deficiency in the West is rare, but diabetes is not. Chromium picolinate is the most commonly recommended form. More recently, GTF chromium has been recommended as better. I found the latter lowered my blood sugar for a week (after the several weeks it takes to work), and then elevated it! Because we all differ, your experience may not be the same.

No medicinal herb has been clinically proven to do what insulin can do. Claims from chiropractors, homeopaths, and hypnotists to cure diabetes are also without much support. Remember that testimonies to cures constitute the least reliable evidence, and only a fool repeatedly duplicates other people's mistakes.

The book *Dr. Rosenfeld's Guide to Alternative Medicine* is a valuable guide in this matter. Over twenty times Dr. Rosenfeld refers to diabetes, but not once does he hail any item from the pharmacopoeia of unorthodox treatments as a "cure," though he suggests a few remedies may help alleviate symptoms.

The author is insightful but charitable as he reviews acupuncture, kinesiology, aromatherapy, ayurveda, bee venom, cell therapy, chelation, chiropractic, craniosacral therapy, enzymes, diet therapy, fasting, herbs, high colonics and coffee enemas, homeopathy, hypnosis, iridology, light therapy, magnetic therapy, neurolinguistic programming, oxygen therapy, and reflexology, etc.

It is important to observe that Dr. Rosenfeld does not reject all of these as quackery. His main contention is that they do not live up to the advertising. He does see some value in chiropractic for some ills, likewise certain herbs including saw palmetto, evening primrose oil, and ginger, etc. Here are typical lines from the discussion on herbal therapy:

> The **good news** about botanicals is that some have been shown to be useful, and they're usually less expensive than pharmaceuticals. Examples of some approved (or at least tolerated) by the traditional medical community include ginger (to prevent motion sickness), garlic (to lower cholesterol and blood pressure), chamomile (to promote sleep and improve digestion), and valerian (a mild sedative).

> The **bad news** about herbal produces is that their production remains unregulated, and there are concerns about their purity and safety.

—p. 167.

Dr. Rosenfeld believes that topically applied "chamomile neutralizes some of the undesirable by-products that are thought to be responsible for complications in diabetics..." (p. 178). A similar recommendation is given to oil of evening primrose.

When Dr. Rosenfeld comes to iridology he is more sweeping. "Iridology does not appear to have any scientific basis, and none of its findings or claims have ever been reproduced" (p. 244).

On homeopathy we read: "…for symptoms that are not life-threatening, and for which conventional medicine has either no treatment or a potentially toxic treatment, homeopathy may be a reasonable alternative" (p. 216).

But going back to diabetes and alternative medicine. Dr. Rosenfeld says that all researchers are agreed that bee venom should not be used for this disease, likewise the cell therapy of Niehans, fasting, homeopathy, and most of the alternative medicine offerings. On the other hand, Dr. Rosenfeld believes chromium supplements may help some diabetics, and that some forms of hydrotherapy may be helpful though not curative. Though not infallible, of course, I recommend this volume as a safeguard against unwarranted hopes and wasted expenditures of time and money.

Possibly the best presentation on herbs for diabetes is found in *The Healing Power of Herbs,* by Michael T. Murray, N.P, (Prima Health), pp. 355 to 362. Dr. Murray discusses studies that have been done on the following herbal possibilities for diabetics: onions and garlic, bitter melon, gymnema sylvestre, fenugreek, salt bush (atriplex), pterocarpus, bilberry, grape seed, and ginkgo biloba.

9

A Response to Issues Raised by a Specialist in Diabetes—Part One

A medical scientist has graciously considered this manuscript and appropriately offered several caveats and suggestions. To these I can but give my opinion as a Christian layman whose interest in preventive medicine for over half a century makes him sensitive to, and grateful for, the matters raised.

There must be zero literature currently on diabetes from the prospective of a Christian with diabetes. Doubtless there is some on cancer but I doubt there is much on chronic non-fatal illnesses. There are several sub-issues here. Firstly, there is the general emotional response to a life-threatening or debilitating illness and how a Christian should respond to that. Behind this emotional response, and giving it a sharp edge, is the threat of aging and death that we all must face even as those who believe in Eternal Life. God alone is immortal. Second, and related, is the more specific issue of how we resolve illnesses that appear to be behavioral, when our behavior has been impeccable. What about the Christian who has inherited a tendency to depression, What went wrong when they get clinically depressed. And what about Pritikin getting leukemia?

—Personal letter to Desmond Ford, August 9, 2000.

The mature Christian remains a sinful human being exposed to the same tendencies to anxiety as the nonChristian. Even Billy Graham confesses, in his recent autobiography *Just as I Am*, a tendency to worry so much that he bites his nails; at the same time he remains aware deep down that God is still in control of things. No wonder then that we lesser Christians must battle with the temptation of the fear of the approach of death. Every problem of life, and every illness great and small, is a mini death. It is because of this fact that they carry such weight.

We see in troubles and illnesses the shadow of ultimate oblivion. What threatens to be an eternal abyss yawns before us. Our blood, at least for a time, runs cold. How should Christians relate to this universal experience?

There are, of course, some very simple approaches. Many have learned to recite the Shepherd's Psalm in times of anxiety. "Yea, though I walk through the valley of the shadow of death, I will fear no evil, for thou art with me." It has been said that there are 365 "fear nots" (or synonyms) in the Bible. That's one for every day of the year. No one can read the Gospels without being touched by the words so frequently found on the lips of Jesus: "Fear not!"; "be of good courage." Hebrews 2:14 tells us that Christ came to deliver us from the fear of death and, as mentioned previously, all our troubles are in a sense mini deaths and bring fear.

Many Christians have devoted themselves to the close study of what the Bible says about trouble and the believer's attitude towards it. At a time when multitudes were dying like flies in London, the famous preacher and poet John Donne found himself threatened with death. As he heard the bells tolling, he wondered if they were tolling for him. It was at this time that he resolutely set himself to studying all that the Scripture had to say about fear. He concluded that there are only two options—to fear God with reverence and love, as he delivers us from all other fears, or to fear every threatening shadow that daily life projects.

Perhaps at a deeper level one needs to be aware of the significance of Christian anthropology—its doctrine concerning the nature of human beings. In essence, it can be summed up as saying that all of us are ignorant, wicked, and mortal. Awareness of these theological truths, which the twentieth century has so adequately demonstrated, is a safeguard and armor for all the battles of life. Because of our ignorance, we all make many mistakes (James 3:2), and because of our mistakes—both intentional and accidental—we fear death.

Men are not afraid that death is the end; they are afraid that death is not the end. "It is appointed unto men once to die, and after that the judgment" (Heb 9:27). The confessions of the ancient myths and philosophy of Egypt, Greece, and Rome help us here. They all testify to the universal conviction that one must give an account for one's misdeeds and that this accounting will take place after death.

I am suggesting that once we really understand the Christian teaching about death we are fortified against "the slings and arrows of outrageous fortune," including organic and debilitating disease, and all the shadows that illnesses cast. The world has many approaches regarding the threat of death, but none of them is adequate. They can warn us against "pie in the sky when you die by and by" and urge us to believe in "one world at a time," further urging that "life can be beautiful." But, as has been recognized by deeper thinkers, life with a dagger in it is not really beautiful. No bouquet with death-dealing fragrance is really beautiful. It is diabolical.

Until the beginning of the twentieth century, until the sinking of the Titanic and the declaration of war in 1914, the theories of human progress were offered to fill the void in the hearts of men. All those hopes have now been dashed by the bloodiest century of all time. We become aware, as George Buttrick said long ago, that "in plain truth history is meaningless unless we can come to some bearable terms with death."

The same writer offers us a summary of popular evasions in the face of death:

> When a man is critically sick, the doctor does not tell him. His friends are likely to assure him, "You look much better today." The minister is advised that it might be wiser if he did not see him: 'He might think he is going to die.' If the minister asks, "well, isn't he, sometime?" the family circulates the word that the church should have a happier-spirited minister. Meanwhile the man's wife searches for insurance policies and the will, perhaps finds neither: he has written none, because he might not think he is going to die. When he does die, the undertaker strives to make it appear that he has not died: he dresses him in a tuxedo and lays him in a narrow box as if he were asleep, even though a man does not usually sleep in a tuxedo in a narrow box. There is a funeral, for, unfortunately for our evasions, the man has died: 'too bad about So-and-So. But let's not think about it!' so we run to our familiar hiding place in the sensate world... In truth, religion alone refuses to be blind to the fact of death.

—*Christ and Man's Dilemma*, Abingdon-Cokesbury Press,
Nashville, New York, 1946, pp. 85-86.

In 2 Timothy 1:10, the believer is told that Christ has abolished death. He is our real strength and refuge. The New Testament further teaches that the moment we believe in the Savior, we have eternal life. See John 5:24 and 1 John 5:11, 12. Eternal life is not something we are only given in the resurrection. We have it now, and its title deed is the imputed righteousness of Christ given freely to all those who trust in the merits of the crucified Savior, the representative of us all.

The counterfeit of this truth is the hope that man naturally has immortality, and that death is just the opening of a gate in a garden wall to admit us into a more beautiful place—more fragrant, more refreshing than anything we have ever known. This view of natural immortality has not worn well with thinkers, philosophers or theologians. Even the nonChristian man often has overwhelming doubts about life after death.

There is an epitaph on a tombstone in the United States that reads as follows:

> Don't bother me now,
> Don't bother me never,
> I want to be dead,
> Forever and ever.

Bernard Shaw has affirmed that he could not endure being George Bernard Shaw forever. And it's probably true that every thoughtful man shrinks from mere continuance of years into eternity. When Moody declared that he had more trouble with himself than any other man he had ever met, he spoke for all of us. Which one of us has not echoed often the cry of the apostle "O wretched man that I am!" (Rom 7:24)? It is our sinfulness that makes immortality unappealing.

The judgement is referred to about a thousand times in the Bible. Every Bible writer brings it into focus. But the wonderful news in the New Testament is that we have the verdict of the Last Judgment the moment we believe in Christ. This Scripture is the essence of justification, the theme elaborated particularly in the book of Romans. See especially Romans 1:16-17; Romans 5:1-19; and 2 Corinthians 5:14-21. Faith in Christ, our representative, and in the great exchange whereby he took our sins to give us his righteousness, is the best defense against fear. See Roman 8:28-39 and share in the triumphant proclamation of the apostle as he rejoices in the fact that neither death nor life nor anything else can separate him from the love of God in Christ.

An elderly Christian who had little education was told by his doctor reluctantly that the issue of his illness was certain to be fatal and that, very shortly, his last day would come. His response to the doctor's pronouncement was: "Don't let that bother you none, Doc; that's the day I've been living for."

To understand the Christian teaching about death more fully, we must recognize that the New Testament nowhere promises a natural extension of life beyond death. We are told to seek for immortality (Rom 2:7), and that God alone has it (1 Tim 6:16). Never does the New Testament present a doctrine of the hereafter that's distinct from the doctrine of the atonement. Mere continuance of life after death would be a curse unless something had been done about the evil of our lives.

In A. J. Cronin's book *The Citadel,* he pictures a young doctor coming to the awful realization that in compromising with his own principles he has brought himself into judgment. When he opened the purse of his recently deceased wife, he found there the clippings of his Galahad days when he fought for the rights of miners and imperiled his own reputation and income. Now, in awful self-recrimination, he cries out, as he thinks of his surrender to greed in his more recent years. "You thought you could get away with it. You thought you were getting away with it. But by God! You weren't."

The fact is that "All have sinned," and all deserve death. No wonder William Tyndale said that the Christian gospel was "good, glad, and merry tidings, that makes the heart to sing and the feet to dance." The gospel tells us that God has done something about our sin, even nailed it to the cross of Christ. As Christ gave his robe, that beautiful robe woven without seam, to his crucifiers, so he offers to us his perfect righteousness despite what we have done to him by lives of selfishness and neglect. It is in the glory of this accomplishment by our Savior that death shrinks and fear dwindles.

I quote again from George Buttrick:

> Death is the final and deepest sign of our ignorance, our finitude and our sin. Immortality would be no comfort, but grievous discomfort, if sin were not overcome. Yet that redemption would be no redemption, but only the pathos of an unfinished symphony, if there were no assurance of eternal life. Christ is Judgement: by him we know why we are troubled in conscience. Christ is Redemption: by him the dread circle of our wickedness is broken. Christ is Resurrection: for our tragic sense of death and life he gives the triumphant promise of life and death—life in his death, and in his victory over death.

—Ibid., p. 104.

We come now to the second point in the chapter's introductory letter—what about illness that appears to be behavioral when our behavior has been impeccable? How can you explain the Christian who inherits a tendency to depression? What happened there?

It is a strange quirk of human nature that we demand to know everything about the origin of our troubles and evils that confront us, and yet we are well aware that, in the majority of matters concerning us, we know almost nothing beyond what is immediately apparent. Was it Einstein who said that the greatest discovery of the twentieth century was that we only know one ten millionth percent about anything? Why should Christians presume to think they could understand all about providence when they know almost nothing about creation?

Even the Christian Bible does not condescend to give us minute instruction about either of these. The early chapters of Genesis are so written under inspiration that they could be taught to the majority of people who through the ages have not even been able to read. It is not an abstract scientific statement, or all we would have would be an equation quite indecipherable to us. And yet it tells us all we actually must know for practical purposes, that we are not an accident but the creation of God. Scripture is similarly reserved about the mystery of suffering.

When Job, the most perfect man in the earth of that day, wrestled with the sickness and troubles that had come upon him, God did not give him a detailed explanation. Instead, God asked him questions about the nature of the realities surrounding him and, at the close of that experience, Job put his hand over his mouth and confessed that he was vile. In his own favorite book, *Till We Have Faces*, C. S. Lewis pictures the insight that comes when God becomes our central focus. Lewis says that, when we are confronted with God, all our questions die away. God himself is the only adequate answer.

A small Christian boy born blind was asked how he could reconcile his blindness with a loving God. He responded: "Even so, Father, for it seemed good in thy sight." Christians must remember the words of Jesus in John 13:7: "What I do thou knowest not now; but thou shalt know hereafter." A major purpose in our ignorance is that we might be cast in dependence upon God and find that courage, zest, and true living that comes from walking the plank constantly with him. Paul reminds us that "We walk by faith, not by sight."

Let us not be discouraged by this. The scientist has to do the same, even though he might be an atheist. He sees the sunset, but knows that it does not set. By faith, he understands about the revolution of the earth. The fact is, none of us know what a single hour or day might bring forth, and therefore we have to live by faith. We do so many things in anticipation of a future that may never transpire. We do so by faith and hope. In fact, all the best things of life that motivate us and keep us going are the invisible things—faith, hope, and love. Who has ever seen these jewels or handled them? They are the invisible realities that undergird all human experience. To live meaningfully by sight alone is not possible.

Furthermore, the Christian must remember that if the impeccable Son of God could cry out on the cross, "My God, My God, Why?" there is nothing strange when the same temptation comes to him or her. It is perfectly natural.

In the last verses of 2 Corinthians chapter 4 and the early verses of chapter 5, Paul reminds us that the approach of death cannot be deferred. He says that we live in decaying bodies, and that weakness is our birthright, but that God has a new body for us, prepared in the heavens, to give us on the resurrection morning. Meanwhile, in the twelfth chapter he reminds us that when we are weak, then are we strong, and he cries out triumphantly, "Most gladly, therefore, will I rather glory in my infirmities, that the power of Christ may rest upon me." (2 Cor 12:9). Paul lived in the strength supplied by the words that come immediately before his confession: "My grace is sufficient for you, for my power is made perfect in weakness." So it must be with every Christian. There will never be a day in our lives when we are not confronted by the specter of evil and disaster. How cheering the words of Ephesians about the shield of faith "…with which you can extinguish all the flaming arrows of the evil one." (Eph 6:16).

It was C. S. Lewis who said that God is never more pleased than when the Christian looks around upon a universe from which every vestige of God seems to have departed, and yet resolves to trust in him. All of us must learn to say with Job, "Though he slay me, yet will I trust in him." You should read 1 Corinthians 15 often. It sets forth the glory of the coming resurrection day, made certain by Christ's own resurrection. Death need hold no terrors for the believing Christian, despite the recurring temptations that come from the great adversary as he attempts to wear down our faith.

Then there is the question about the Christian's relationship to medicine and therapies. "What then about the treatment? There is a need to develop a rationale to support a unique approach for treatment if one is Christian. If our bodies are the temple of God, how would treatment strategies change?"

Christians in philosophy and science have long pointed out that there would have been no Western science but for monotheism—the faith offered by Judaism and Christianity. Even Islam is dependent upon that revelation, as found in the early books of the Old Testament and accepted by the Koran. Prior to the acceptance of belief in a single omnipotent, omniscient, omnipresent God, everything was the creature of chance, as the reading of all ancient Greek stories makes clear. To the ancient Greek, anything could happen at any time, at any place. There was no such thing as natural, invariable, reliable law. All was fluid. But the Christian monotheistic view inherited from Judaism, itself the fruit of revelation, has changed all that. Christians therefore rejoice in all the abilities of science to mitigate human ills.

While we mourn that science has often been abused, resulting in death-dealing inventions, we thank God for the marvelous discoveries in his providence that have wiped out infectious diseases and, through the principles of sanitation, increased longevity. Seeing in all truth, including scientific truth, the gift of God, the Christian will wish to avail himself or herself of the very best that medical science has to offer. But though we call it a science, in many respects medicine is still an art. The orthodoxy of today may be the heterodoxy of tomorrow and vice versa. There have been hundreds of short-lived therapies, once hailed as breakthroughs, and later found as devastating instruments.

Two million women in USA were given DES as a protection against miscarriage, though all the evidence pointed against this risky procedure. Cancer has sadly resulted for hundreds, perhaps thousands, because of this medical error, and many children of the women treated are also developing cervical cancer. The introduction to an early edition of Harrison's *Principles of Internal Medicine* should never be forgotten. There the warning was given that the physician must remember that all therapeutic remedies have a price tag attached. Actually it is the principles of hygiene, rather than the marvelous discoveries of medicine, that have added so much to our life span. But we must never lessen the significance of the marvelous discoveries made by pioneers in the field of medicine. All should be hailed with gratitude, and there should be no reluctance to avail oneself of the best medical science.

However, when the experts differ, the layman is left free to choose. And in many areas of medical science, including even therapies for diabetes, the experts are not agreed. The ADA has reversed itself more than once. The latest instance is its withdrawal of the dogma that diabetics should include in their diet approximately 65 percent of carbohydrates.

Anecdotal evidence is of the least value, and yet personal experience is hard to gainsay. Christians have often used the old saying: "A person with an experience is not at the mercy of a person who only has an argument." All scientific hypotheses are tested by the empirical approach. Do they work? Are they successful in accomplishing what they set out to do? Is more harm done than good by the therapy?

The therapy for diabetes has reversed itself repeatedly. Anyone who reads the history can see that quite clearly. In the nineteen century, people with diabetes were starved—and actually starved to death. Later, with the awareness it is carbohydrates that raise blood sugars, came the warning to eat little of carbohydrates, but that resulted in consumption of animal products *ad nauseam*, and consequent heart disease in epidemic proportions. So again the therapy was changed.

Let us not seem to bypass the marvelous discovery of insulin by Best and Banting which has saved millions of lives. But now many researchers are asking whether even insulin therapy in some instances can do unwarrantable damage. Which is not to deny for a moment that millions are and ever will be dependent upon insulin. Recent caveats are just suggesting that care must be used even with this wonderful modality.

For decades the emphasis has been on carbohydrate consumption of up to about 65 percent in the diet, but in the last decade or so, many warnings have come from individual investigators regarding this approach. There now seems to be considerable evidence that there may be a better therapy than a high consumption of carbohydrate for some sufferers with diabetes. As I have read the literature, it seems to me that there is considerable evidence that a diet high in monounsaturates, rather than overt carbohydrates, could be useful to a large proportion of diabetics. Of course, I do not here refer to type 1 diabetes. And it must be said also that while there is great good sense in stressing exercise as an invisible insulin, it must be remembered that many diabetics are not physically able to pursue vigorous exercise.

The stress earlier in this manuscript has been that the diabetic above all people needs to exercise self-discipline, and that the Christian has the best motivation to that end. This self-discipline should be manifested in caring for all the habits of life that have impact upon behavior and health. Obviously, the believer needs to repudiate gluttony and sloth. Abstemiousness and the temperate employment of one's physical and mental abilities should characterize all those who have faith in Christ. The Christian who has refused the allurement of alcohol and tobacco must also learn to refuse the allurements of refined carbohydrates and, perhaps, even large amounts of unrefined carbohydrates if they are not contributory to his or her health.

So much of life appears to be a matter of balance. Too many have emphasized diet and forgotten exercise, while many have emphasized exercise and forgotten diet. Both approaches are wrong. We are what we eat, and they never bury anything that moves. Both of these axioms are true.

On the other hand, there are genetic factors. In some instances, obesity is genetic, and likewise with many other things that tend to illness, and diabetes in particular. A Christian is responsible for doing what he or she can do, not for what he or she can't do. To whom much is given, much is expected, but to whom little is given, little is expected.

The issue of medications is one that must be weighed very carefully. The book *Cured to Death* by scientific authors of good repute should be included in one's survey of the evidence. See also *The Confessions of a Medical Heretic*, a volume that may be extreme in some positions, but is worthy of attention because of the qualifications of its author. See also *Matters of Life and Death* by Eugene D. Robin. There is no question that hundreds of thousands of people the world around die annually because of pharmaceuticals unwisely prescribed or used. It's just as certain that a far greater number have found benefit from pharmaceuticals rightly prescribed and applied.

As the editor of the book *Principles of Medicine* has reminded us, every prescription has a price tag attached. Benefits must be weighed against dangers and losses. However, when we come to insulin itself, it is not really in the identical position of many pharmaceuticals. It mimics the body's own creation, provides a life-saving solution for multitudes. None should hesitate to use it if it is the best therapy for their particular need. Indeed, in many cases, it is the only appropriate therapy. No Christian should fail to thank God for insulin, if that is the nearest and best medication for their diabetes. Yet all this will be done with the awareness that even insulin has its problems.

As pointed out elsewhere in this manuscript, there are rare instances where some people have died from the unwise use of insulin as they have suffered an episode of hypoglycemia in their sleep. To sleep alone for some diabetics may be dangerous. There are now many voices that are saying the indiscriminate use of insulin in excessive amounts may contribute to heart disease and other problems. A Christian who is neither a scientist nor a qualified physician, needs help in making decisions about such matters. An intelligent Christian physician is worth his or her weight in gold many times over, and should be resorted to with gratitude and prayer by the believer.

Too often Christians can climb mountains, but have difficulty with stones in their shoes. Even believers can often make grave mistakes because of little things that can be simply remedied. The matter of using a glucose monitor, or inserting insulin needles, falls into this category. I personally hate the sight of blood and could never be a physician. The first pricking of my finger for the glucose monitor was done with extreme reluctance. Now I do it after thousands of times without even thinking about it. The same is true for the use of insulin needles. It becomes second nature and is no more a trial than blowing one's nose.

The issue of the Christian's attitude to alternative medicine has also been raised. In response I can but give my opinion that to those who read widely, the evidence seems very clear indeed that much of alternative medicine engages in hyperbole rather than truth. Its dependence on anecdotal evidence, for example, in many cases leaves it open to severe criticism. Which is not to say for a moment, that no good can be found in this arena. The respected physician and author Dr. Isadore Rosenfeld has written the book entitled *Guide to Alternative Medicine*. In it he warns against many forms of therapy in this field, but recommends others. In some instances he says: "Give it a trial." Probably his approach is the one most warranted by modern knowledge—alternative medicine is to be viewed with care and a measure of skepticism, but also with the awareness that much that is now orthodoxy was once an alternative therapy.

This manuscript has given quotations from respected medical leaders to the effect that there is no herbal treatment for diabetes scientifically proven to be effective. The same is true of other alternative approaches to diabetes. But I do not regard the stress on monounsaturates as a dubious form of alternative medicine, for many researchers have validated this new approach.

As pointed out earlier, probably half a million scientific papers have been presented on diabetes, and many of them are worthless. So again the issue arises—how does the Christian deal with this mass of scientific data? I have suggested above what I consider to be the right approach. To thank God for medical science, and to seek out with gratitude informed and responsible physicians, competent in the area of diabetic therapies. But as we can surrender our conscience to no man entirely, so all sufferers with diabetes should endeavor, as they are able, to weigh conflicting opinions, and then experiment for themselves.

I recognize the dangers in this approach, but submit that there are equal or greater dangers in any other approach. This is in view of the constantly changing face of diabetic therapy; in view of a rather wide spread misinterpretation of the DCCT trial (according to some who were actually present at those meetings), according to the history of failure in diabetic therapy for decades, in view of the fact that the majority of diabetics over a long period ultimately develop complications, in view of the incomplete nature of human knowledge—in view of all these things, a measure of skepticism is warranted, and even desirable, in this medical field, as in all others.

None should forget the thousands of people who die every year because of unnecessary surgeries. We should remember that millions are hospitalized annually around the world because of drugs that should not have been prescribed or have been prescribed and applied wrongly. Hospitals are dangerous places like war zones, to be avoided where possible, but accepted with great gratitude when clearly necessary. Iatrogenic and nosocomial diseases (caused by doctors and hospitals) are a major source of death in all countries of the world today. Because of these facts, and many similar ones, the Christian must walk with care and prayer.

None can hope to encompass all the scientific data on diabetes. Not even the specialist can do that. Its seems important to distinguish the princes from the paupers among the authors. It seems also wise to view the present in the light that shines from history. A well-known book was entitled *A History of Some Scientific Blunders,* but a much larger book could be written on the history of medical blunders. Despite these seemingly negative warnings, I would stress that I believe there is no man more worthy of higher acclaim and appreciation than the intelligent Christian physician who has given both his heart and head to medical problems, and truly lives by the Hippocratic oath and the Christian faith.

A principle worthy of consideration is that the best often becomes the worst. As Shakespeare said, "Lilies fester worse than weeds." Woman, according to the creation story, was the apex of God's creative work. However, as the highest, she can fall the lowest. Religion is both necessary and saving, but there is nothing worse in the entire world than bad religion. The greater the potentiality of something for good, the greater the danger that, when abused or misused, it can yield evil.

What is true of religion and of science in general is true of medicine in particular. God has worked in the field of medicine and has inspired countless men and women of research in practical fields. God is in the business of helping people physically, as well as spiritually, and he has worked through modern medicine to that end. But as surely as science has often invented instruments of destruction as well as labor saving devices, so in the science of medicine dangers exist, and must be recognized. I take the liberty of repeating the maxim that, where experts disagree, the layman must make his or her choice.

10

A Response to Issues Raised by a Specialist in Diabetes—Part Two

One medical reviewer of this manuscript has written some thoughtful words regarding the methods of medicine at its best.

I quote:

A catch cry of modern medicine is "evidence." Modern medicine believes it can no longer rely on expert opinion. Expert opinion is gathered by long experience, but our memories that create the current viewpoint are flawed and biased by all sorts of things. In short, it is limited by human frailty. Expert opinion is an extension of anecdotal evidence. Anecdotal evidence can lead to discovery, but its use as evidence is necessarily limited. Nonetheless, personal experience refines global evidence and so has validity on one level. Moreover, opinion needs to be backed by direct not theoretical evidence. Admittedly, the evidence is not always available, but the goal is a good and right one.

—Personal letter to Desmond Ford, August 9, 2000.

Here warning comes from the scientific parallel to the two mythical rocks that threatened ancient Greek mariners. Unless I exercise great care, I may be wrecked on one rock or the other. One can take the risk of being ahead of contemporary medical judgments, or pursue the less dangerous but still risky course of being the last to adopt newly discovered vital evidence. But temperaments, classified as "liberal" and "conservative," each have their problems.

Let us consider this matter of evidence. Those who have investigated the contributions of epistemology are aware that absolute proof about anything in the real world is not available to us. It would require (1) perfect measuring instruments; (2) an infinite number of observations; (3) perfect objectivity. None of

56

these three is available to human investigators. The only place for absolute proof is when we scribble on a plain surface, as a blackboard, putting the equivalent of the left-handed side of an equation on the right side using other figures or symbols. So perfection of evidence will never be available to us in this life.

Courts of law have long recognized this fact. Thus in a case involving a sentence of life and death, the verdict must be based upon evidence beyond any reasonable doubt, whereas in civil cases there need be merely a preponderance of evidence. Because, as epistemology again reminds us, all thought operates on the basis of nonprovable, intuitive axioms, there are obvious limitations to all ventures of human reflection and investigation. Human frailty can often mar the quality of evidence presented. For example, it is a highly dangerous procedure to go too far ahead of one's peers in the medical profession. It could mean the losing of one's medical license and the privilege of helping one's fellow men in an official capacity.

On the other hand, the history of medicine is replete with examples of men who risked their reputation on what they felt was considerable evidence pointing to a new direction. Louis Pasteur and the renowned Dr. Sammelweis contended against medical prejudice in their day and ventured ahead of their fellows to the great blessing of the human race. It seems so strange to us now that medical professionals could have examined new patients with unwashed hands for decades, but such was indeed the case. And when criticism of this procedure was leveled, it aroused a hue and cry, which shortened life for some conscientious researchers. Nevertheless, but for the reluctance of the medical profession to quickly embrace new approaches, tremendous harm could be wrought by supposed "cures" or novel procedures.

Another example of the dangers brought to us by human frailty is the matter of the accepted therapy for breast cancer over four score years. Radical mastectomies, radiation, and chemical approaches have been used for nearly a century with very limited success. According to some researchers, these modalities have resulted in great harm in hundreds of thousands of cases. Some modern researchers now tell us that the original conclusions regarding the right therapies for breast cancer were not based on correctly structured experiments. Journal articles in recent decades—in the *Lancet*, and *the New England Journal of Medicine*, and other medical publications—have warned against radical mastectomies. In most cases these are both unnecessary and harmful. Similarly, the benefits of radiation and chemotherapy, it is now being suggested, have been overexaggerated. This is not to deny that each of these therapies has an appropriate role for some patients.

Only in one instance have I given unqualified support for a diabetes reference work (*Textbook on Diabetes*, by Pickup and Williams). It seems to me that this particular textbook is more thoroughly based on available evidence than the others I have quoted. It also seems less biased than most of the other volumes. However, there is a more recent work on diabetes called *Clinical Diabetes Mellitus*, edited by John K. Davidson, M.D., Ph.D., which was published in 2000. This almost one-thousand-page book is very thoroughly documented by leaders in the field of diabetes. A highly esteemed academic diabetologist, Davidson worked with Dr. Best (the co-discoverer of insulin therapy) from 1960 to 1965. He was not only a student but also, ultimately, an assistant and associate professor of physiology from 1965 to 1968.

Davidson says of that experience: "Charley and his colleagues taught me how to do research, how to teach, and how to provide excellent clinical care to those who have diabetes mellitus." (p. v.). Dr. Davidson is Professor of Medicine Emeritus of Emory University School of Medicine, and Founding Director of the Diabetes Unit, at Grady Memorial Hospital, in Atlanta, Georgia. This most up-to-date, carefully researched volume is a good example of the need to avoid echoing former theories just because they have been acceptable to medical science in past decades.

One needs to keep in mind that most books in the nonfiction field are "echo" books, containing very little original thinking or original research. This volume, while highly orthodox in approximately 98 percent of its pages, is quite unorthodox in its chapter on "Oral Agents in the Treatment of Diabetes Mellitus." I do not mean that the presentation of this topic is entirely new in its approach or content but it is very much in the forefront by its emphases. From the most well-known reference work in medicine, the *Merck Manual*, to the most recent tiny volumes on the subject of diabetes, it is assumed that oral agents for diabetes are not only an acceptable approach for millions, but the natural course of recommendation if diet and exercise fail. This book, however, goes way beyond that status quo.

Having personally read about fifty discussions on sulfonylureas in recent years, I found the one that has just appeared in Dr. Davidson's textbook *(Clinical Diabetes Mellitus)* to be staggering, invigorating, and enlightening. The presentation is well in advance of the vast majority of sources about orthodox treatments. While it is true that some of these sources give warnings about the use of sulfonylureas, I have not found such stringent condemnation of the typical medical laxity in prescribing such for millions of sufferers around the world. Because of our desire to stress both the necessity for basing conclusions on adequate evidence, and also the wisdom of refusing to be "an echo" of the status quo, I append points from this chapter as illustrations.

In the splendid chapter "Oral Agents in the Treatment of Diabetes Mellitus," Doctors Michael Berger and Bernard Richter make the following points:

• The safety of oral antidiabetic medications has never been proven. Their almost universal use is the result of commercial and political pressures.

• Pharmaceutical manufacturers have a greater say than the medical profession in the matter of the use of these oral pills.

• The potential risk of prolonged use of these medications is considerable. And their usage should be restricted. Not one of them has yet been thoroughly tested.

• In the late 70s, certain of these widely-used pills were banned as a result of overwhelming evidence that they were life-threatening.

• The marketing campaigns promoting these expensive medications are unparalleled.

• The main danger for diabetics is coronary heart disease (CHD), and no evidence has been provided that the pills lessen this danger. Indeed they raise LDLs and have other damaging effects.

• While Medline between 1966 and 1997 pointed to 8,824 publications promoting these drugs, it referred to only two studies that warned against them, despite the fact that the conclusions of these two have never been refuted, though often criticized unfairly.

Sulfonylurea therapy results in ischemic damage to the myocardium and therefore increases cardiovascular mortality. Hypertension, a major problem for most diabetics, is also a problem. This therapeutic approach is actually one of carelessness and laziness.

The authors quote from Dr. John Rollo who wrote the following, 200 years ago:

> We have to lament that our mode of cure is so contrary to the inclination of the sick. Though perfectly aware of the efficacy of the (diet) regimen, and the impropriety of deviations, yet they commonly trespass, concealing what they feel as a transgression on themselves. They express a regret that a medicine

could not be discovered, however nauseous or distasteful, which would suppress the necessity of any restriction of diet.

Where dietary and exercise regimens fail, insulin is preferable to diabetic pills. Those who choose the latter take considerable risks.

I doubt if there is any example in recently published literature on diabetes so strongly indicting carelessness with regard to the prescription of oral tablets for diabetes. Note that I have already said that the warnings sounded in this chapter have appeared elsewhere. But in the majority of discussions of oral pills, the warnings do not find a prominent place.[1] In this recent book, *Clinical Diabetes Mellitus*, we have a fine example of the need for care in weighing medical evidence. The status quo may not be right. "Echo" books are often only worthy of a glance.

It may be a matter for considerable regret that a vast number of people who have written on diabetes have not themselves suffered from the particular affliction. Far from being a malevolent remark, this statement is pleading the case for the millions of diabetics whose counselors have not always been activated by the conviction of the life and death urgency of their work. "Only the wounded can minister to the wounded."

In case I am misunderstood, the opposite side of the picture must be emphasized. The ideal and the real rarely match. Every physician's heartache and perplexity is the stumbling block of the human nature of the typical patient. Few are willing to be drastically change their habits and, because of the strength of lifelong habits, they are psychologically unable to do so. And there are multitudes whose genetic inheritance makes the issue of weight control quite distinct from the simple practices open to the naturally lean. Pills do have their appropriate place.

Earlier I warned against the vast majority of alternative medical approaches. There is insufficient evidence to substantiate the widespread use of any of these for diabetes. So the burden of these last pages is certainly not intended to move the reader from confidence in established medical practice to a greater confidence in alternative medical approaches. Again to quote one correspondent: "I believe there is a plant (Akeefruit, Blighia Sapida) that will bring glucose down but is otherwise quite toxic." Most local bookstores carry a book on the topic of poisonous garden plants. See also *The Use and Safety of Common Herbs and Herbal Teas*, by Dr. Winston Craig, published by Golden Harvest Books, Berrien Springs, Michigan.

The quotations I have used in this manuscript have been offered not in valida-
tion of the entire contents of the works cited, but because of light offered on a
particular point. Because I believe that the evidence is overwhelmingly in favor of
a vegetarian or even a vegan diet, I have considerable difficulty with the diet suggested by many popular writers on this topic.

Nothing in this little book questions for one moment the validity of the scientific method in its place. The only compelling evidence in medical matters is
arrived at by the prospective, doubled-blinded, placebo-controlled, randomized
clinical trial. Otherwise bias and misleading intuitions after limited experience
can give credit to dangerous errors. Every diabetic must do his or her best to
avoid both extremes. They must keep in mind that medicine is indeed an art
rather than a science when strictly considered, for there is much more to learn
than has yet been learned. Many of the breakthroughs hailed in the media as
great advances for medicine, prove not to be when tested by time. Phenacetin was
used for decades to the detriment of millions of people all around the world, and
only in our own lifetime has its dangers been revealed by the same medical community that endorsed it for so long. The Harvard Medical School and other
authorities have told us recently that even one of the worst of former diabetic vil-
lains, the egg, may not be quite as bad as it was once thought. It is now recognized that the fat in the egg is unsaturated, and therefore the impact of the
cholesterol may not be as severe as indicated by the literature of recent decades.
Ultimately, having read widely and prayed much, the diabetic must cautiously
experiment on him or herself. Simultaneously, he or she should be counseling
with a medical specialist whose mind is open to new ideas, but who is nonetheless
respected in his or her field.

I repeat, the books cited in this volume are not endorsed in their entirety. This
present work is a record of one diabetic who for very practical reasons has done
what he could by reading the research and speaking with specialists. This book
makes no claim to be exhaustive in its presentation of the scientific or dietetic
issues. However, the practical essence of all that is known about nutrition can be
summed up in these words: "Eat fresh, whole (that is unrefined and unprocessed
foods), chiefly of vegetable origin." It is not necessary to get a degree in dietetics.
This simple formula will suffice for most intelligent people.

Christianity puts a great deal of stress on the saving nature of faith. It's not
that faith in itself saves, but it is the instrument that lays hold upon the Savior.
Nevertheless, because of the doctrine of original sin, Christianity also warns every
believer against too high a degree of faith in human beings and their theories. In
our modern age one must be a careful, intelligent skeptic in order to survive. Not

all that is old is true gold, but it's also true that if something is absolutely new, it's rarely true.

I advocate wide study of the literature as far as one is able to grapple with the technicalities, and, even more importantly, to have regular recourse to an esteemed medical expert in the area. Above all, there must be constant care and prayer regarding one's own practices and conclusions.

This book is one man's testimony to his experience with this disease, which is the most rapidly growing disease in the twenty-first century. It is a result of the study of hundreds of volumes and articles, but what are they in so vast a field of published literature? It is also the result of personal experimentation. I have found a way (not, of course, devised by me) to keep my blood sugar levels within reasonable figures without endangering my health. I use the following:

- Fresh uncooked vegetables (avoiding those that are overtly carbohydrate, such as potatoes, corn, etc.), I include tomatoes, which don't put my blood sugar up, even though they are considered a fruit.

- Some cooked vegetables (such as eggplant, spinach, and broccoli).

- A lot of soya beans.

- A more moderate quantity of nuts, including peanuts, which are strictly a legume.

- Some eggs and cheese.

Along with this dietetic approach, I exercise vigorously every day, usually for about an hour to one-and-a-half hours [each meal], some time after a meal has lapsed (exercising immediately after a meal affects the blood sugar adversely in my case).

I trust that all readers will recognize that this book makes no claim to being a comprehensive guide to the study of diabetes. It is an endeavor to help thinking Christians facing this challenging disorder in a practical way.

Footnotes

1. One writer who does protest with great vigor against the use of oral medication is Dr. Julian M. Whitaker, in his book *Reversing Diabetes*. Since writing the book, Dr. Whitaker has reversed his position on the advocacy of a high-carbohydrate component in the diabetic diet, but he has not reversed his position against the thoughtless use of pills for diabetics.

While recognizing the necessity for insulin for many diabetics, even here he sounds some warnings, pointing out that over 90 percent of diabetics on insulin have hypoglycemic episodes. I quote:

> "Up to 16 percent reported having an attack at least once a month. Each year about 25 percent of insulin users will have a severe reaction—severe being defined as requiring assistance from another person or requiring hospitalization.

> "In another study of 100 patients, 55 percent had become comatose from severe hypoglycemic reactions. This complication of insulin therapy accounts for about 3 to 7 percent of deaths in the insulin-treated diabetic, and it surely has led to brain damage in a much higher percentage. Hypoglycemia is the rule, not the exception, in insulin-treated diabetics, and it represents a serious threat." (p.102)

On page 113, Dr. Whitaker makes this confession:

> "What continues to plague those of us who treat diabetic patients is that the complications for this disease have never been shown significantly reduced by improved control of the glucose either with insulin or with the oral drugs…Insulin can only do so much, but we continue to expect them single-handedly to lead us to the Promised Land." (pp. 113-114)

This first comment may no longer be true as regards type 1 diabetics, but it may still apply to many type 2 sufferers. We should keep in mind that more than nine out of ten diabetics are type 2 and not type 1.

Dr. Whitaker points out that the results of the famous University Group Diabetes Program show that, despite the efficacy of insulin in accomplishing better glucose control for patients, there were no significant differences in the death rate or the complication rate between the patients so apparently advantaged and others who were not. The *Harvard Health Letter,* July 7, 1988, quotes the same study regarding the use of oral drugs and says: "No convincing scientific data has emerged to refute the original findings." The UGTD researchers concluded that their findings provided no evidence that insulin or any other drug-lowering blood glucose levels altered the course of vascular complications in type 2 diabetes.

But it is with the oral drugs that Dr. Whitaker is most concerned in his book. He quotes a volume produced by the Public Citizens Health Group of Washington DC entitled, *Off Diabetes Pills, A Diabetic's Guide to Longer Life.* Here is a portion of Dr. Whitaker's quotation from this book:

"Warning! Anti-Diabetic Pills Are Dangerous to Your Health.
Stop taking antidiabetic pills as soon as you can;
Go on a diet and lose weight;
Stop seeing your present doctor unless he or she
Genuinely tries to help you lose weight and agrees to
Switch you to insulin if you still have diabetic symptoms
At or below your ideal weight.
These steps could mean the difference between life and death."

—Reversing Diabetes, p.121.

Dr. Whitaker further comments:

"The rapid and widespread acceptance of oral drugs reflects the tunnel vision of many physicians who assume that all diabetic complications will be eliminated if the blood sugar level can be reduced by any means, regardless of other effects the drug has on the body." *(Ibid.,* p.123)

Dr. Whitaker waxes warm as he discusses the reactions to the UGDP study:

"When the UGDP results became public, tens of millions of dollars were being spent on the oral diabetic medications. If primary care physicians across the country were to immediately stop prescribing the oral drugs and intensify efforts of diet and exercise instead, the drug companies sharing in the revenues generated by the oral diabetic drugs would be severely crippled. It is not surprising that the drug companies went to work immediately to cast as much doubt as they could on the conclusions of the UGDP study. They were unbelievably successful. Physicians have never stopped using the drugs. Even today, fifteen years later, they are still prescribing these drugs that might be associated with several thousand unnecessary deaths a year in the diabetic population.

"Today, most physicians honestly believe that the UGDP results were inaccurate. No fault in the design or conduct of the study can be found to support these beliefs"

—Ibid., p. 125.

Dr. Whitaker then proceeds to give evidence regarding the hundreds of thousands of unnecessary deaths caused by the oral drugs and also evidence supporting the UGDP study and refuting its critics.

Our own opinion after reviewing the literature on this subject is that the pills still have a place for some type 2 diabetics, but that they are too commonly and carelessly prescribed as a rule. The multiplying warnings against their cavalier use should be heeded. Otherwise, multitudes will die prematurely.

11

A Word about the Future

This is the best time in the history of the world to have diabetes. Everywhere around the world researchers are feverishly working to find better ways to treat and, perhaps one day even cure, this malady.

It will not be long before the use of lancets is old-fashioned, and diabetics will wear an insulin "watch," which will tell them at any time the state of their blood glucose. And it may only be a few years before many diabetics will have inserted under their armpits a tiny miraculous therapeutic aid, which will both measure glucose continually and inject the required insulin. No more "hypos."

Remember the words of John Wesley. "The best of all is that God is with us."

"If God spared not his own Son, but delivered him up for us all, how shall he not with him also freely give us all things?" (Rom 8:32)

APPENDIX A

Facts About Diabetes

Secondary diabetes can come from pancreatic diseases, which can surface in alcoholics, people with hormone abnormalities like Cushing's Syndrome, or drug or chemically-induced diabetes, those using steroids like prednisone and cortisone, and those with certain genetic syndromes. Antiinflammatories and blood pressure tablets can also cause the blood sugar to rise high and contribute to type 2 diabetes.

There is a relationship between poverty and diabetes also. There are more diabetics among those in the lower social scale.

It's important to remember that there are no absolute guarantees regarding the onset of complications. There are people who exercise rigorous blood sugar control who still get complications, while there are others who seem very careless and get away scot-free. This, however, is a minority fringe, and, for the most part, those who lead disciplined lives in every respect have a far greater chance of remaining healthy all their days.

Cutting back on food intake immediately reduces insulin levels. Many so-called type 2 diabetics can reverse the disease by reducing their caloric intake, losing weight, choosing foods with care, and regularly exercising. Some people in Japan claim to have reversed their diabetes by walking six miles a day.

Exercise cannot control blood glucose though it does influence it. Diet remains the main factor in controlling glucose levels.

It should not be thought that the use of insulin puts an end to all problems. The great danger in insulin is hypoglycemia when the blood sugar dips too low. This can lead to irritability and even coma. If a hypoglycemic attack takes place at nighttime, and the diabetic is alone, there is even the possibility of death, though it is rare.

Insulin is usually used for all type 1 diabetics, but only as a last resort for type 2 diabetics. The patient who uses insulin has a constant balancing act on his or her hands—one must avoid eating too much or too little, and even exercising too much. While insulin has saved millions of lives since its first employment in 1922, it has also taken some lives when used injudiciously.

The same caveat needs to be offered regarding the use of diabetic pills. These also are not a guarantee that one can eat and live as one likes. Self-discipline is still required. Diabetic pills can bring on hypogiycemia if not used with care. Furthermore, none of them are free from possible side effects, and in rare cases some of these effects have proved lethal. Rezulin has been taken off the market recently because it has been responsible for at least 60 known deaths. For every medication there is a price tag attached. All sorts of drugs can be gratefully used, but only as a last resort. For many diabetics the pills cease to work after about five years; in some cases, the wearied pancreas having been thus long provoked to extraordinary effort ultimately signals its exhaustion.

Let not the reader feel discouraged, for many of the most influential people in our world have been diabetics. H.G. Wells and Mary Tyler Moore are just two of the better known ones, but they exist in abundance and shine in every area: for instance, politics, science, education, athletics and the church.

Only a fraction of diabetics continue long on diet therapy alone. **About two-thirds of diabetics are on insulin. Most of the remainder are on tablets.** Nonetheless, it is a great advantage to be able to persevere with the strategy of diet. It avoids many worries and can preserve life for a longer period than medication.

Because every person is different, it is impossible to predict whether, how, and when diabetic complications may arise. In many cases they will never arise. Type 2 diabetes is more linked to heart disease and strokes than eye troubles, whereas with type 1, eye troubles are frequent after 10 years or more, or even earlier in some cases.

One gram of carbohydrate elevates the blood glucose by 3, 4 or 5 points for people who weight 200 lbs., 150 lbs., and 100 lbs., respectively. The life-long risk of amputation of the lower limbs is 5 to 10 percent among diabetics. In almost all cases the amputees are persistent smokers.

Glucose meters are a wonderful invention and a lifesaver for multiple thousands of diabetics. But they are fallible to a degree and can often can give a result of up to 20 too high or too low. They are still valuable regardless. Meters and strips should not be exposed to heat, or to moisture, and a perfectionist may wish to have two different types of meters to check irregular readings for himself. Don't smear blood on the strip, or the reading will be false.

The use of alcohol can raise blood sugar and decrease the body's ability to use its own insulin. Regarding some habits, the diabetic, more than other people, has reason to say, "If in doubt, leave it out."

It is normal for blood sugar to rise after a meal but it should not rise excessively. Once the blood sugar number reaches 250, the diabetic is in the realm of hyperglycemia, and, ideally, the numbers should remain on a 2-hour reading at 180 or less.

The symptoms of hyperglycemia rarely occur unless the blood sugar level is consistently above 250.

It is vital to remember that diabetes is a heterogeneous disorder, and it has many causes. Insulin resistance of the cells, as a result of obesity, is probably the most common cause. Not only the cause, but the course of diabetic complications, is still little understood. Rarely does anyone have all the complications, and often neuropathies take precedence. The complications in general usually take years to develop—the most serious often requiring about 20 to 30 years.

About one-fifth of diabetics escape all visible complications even after having the disease for 40 to 50 years. For most diabetics, after 30 years there is some degree of retinopathy. Often for years that disease itself is quite mild. Seven percent of patients become blind after 30 years. (That figure was offered in the 1980s, but the situation is now better because of laser treatment.)

Any condition that affects the pancreas can cause diabetes. There are a number of adrenal disorders that can cause large amounts of cortisol to enter the bloodstream and raise blood sugar. The body is a very finely-tuned instrument in which all the hormones play their part. We hear much about insulin, but the others also have their place in understanding diabetes. The hormone glucogen, which is also produced by the pancreas, stimulates the liver's production of glucose, but insulin is simultaneously hindered and unable to do its task. Leptin insufficiency, in some instances, can also put "brakes" on insulin efficacy. Thyroid disorders are often found in tandem with type 1 diabetes.

The pancreas is a wonderful factory bringing forth many marvelous products. It houses 100,000 cell clusters known as the islets of Langerhans, which produce insulin. The majority of type 2 diabetics are overweight, and by their obesity have damaged the islets of Langerhans, or made the cells of their body impervious to the insulin produced in the pancreas. But many overweight sufferers can reverse diabetes by losing weight and adopting a new life-style.

It must be confessed that the mechanism of insulin resistance is not yet fully understood. There is a great deal more to learn about diabetes than that we already know. The person who lives temperately and wisely by nature's laws does not need to understand all the mysteries of the body in order to live healthfully. Apparent accidents of time and chance overtake everybody, but obedience to the laws of nature is like slanting the odds in life's gamble. The analogy better suits unbelievers than believers, but it makes the necessary point.

It is perfectly normal for diabetics in their first years with the disease to be tempted with discouragement many, many times. Only hundreds of tests with the monitor can give assurance regarding what foods and how much of them to eat. One learns that sudden elevations mean little. It is only when blood sugar elevations remain high for hours that there is real cause for concern. The diabetic needs courage to face the multiple shocks the monitor renders, but courage, like wisdom and righteousness, is God's gift to those who trust in Christ. Yet it pays to add knowledge to faith.

The symptoms of type 1 and type 2 diabetes are the same—increased hunger and thirst, increased urination, inexplicable fatigue, blurred vision, burning sensations or tingling in the extremities, a multiplying number of infections, slow healing of wounds, and sexual impotence. The disease has developed considerably, but not irreversibly, by the time these symptoms begin to be felt. Often the type 2 sufferer has no symptoms for many years.

For blood sugar tests revealing 140 or above while fasting on two successive occasions, the diagnosis is diabetes. In recent years, many endocrinologists prefer the figure of 126 for safety's sake. The severer, stricter figure can give a diagnosis years earlier, and thus help to avoid complications.

Within approximately five years from diagnosis, most type 2 diabetics seek additional help outside the therapy of diet. Pills are the next step, and five years or more after that, insulin. But remember that there are many diabetics alive today who have been on insulin for more than 50 years and remain in good health.

According to the People's Medical Society, in their recent volume *Understanding Diabetes*, women who do not take ERT (estrogen replacement therapy) at menopause are five times more likely to develop type 2 diabetes. This position on estrogen and diabetes is totally opposite to the position taken two decades ago. Then, having diabetes was considered a contraindication for taking estrogen. But the increased risk of heart disease in diabetic women caused researchers to rethink their position on estrogen.

There are risks with hormonal therapy, and every person must intelligently consider and weigh the benefits against the possible losses. Most researchers today are saying that the danger of heart disease for women is far greater than that of breast cancer, and that hormonal therapy helps to ward off heart disease. Here again, the last word has not yet been spoken. It's because the best of us are still so ignorant, that divine guidance is a personal necessity.

Half of the amputations performed in the United States of America are done on diabetics, and a quarter of the kidney failures in this country are those of diabetics, and the same class has more than twice the risk of heart attack and stroke. Efforts at prevention before diabetes strikes, and vigilance afterwards, are amply rewarded.

Type 1 diabetics fight the harder battle because it usually lasts longer. But in both groups severe complications rarely come before at least 15 years and more often after 20 or even 30 years. Type 1 diabetics have more eye troubles, and type 2 diabetics have more heart disease and strokes.

The further a food is from its natural state, the more likely it is to speedily raise the blood glucose level. Raw foods are to be preferred to cooked, but there is little harm in moderate cooking of vegetables in small amounts.

It is natural for endocrinologists to be wary about challenging the traditional high-carbohydrate diet for diabetics. Whistleblowers are usually not welcome, and old traditions die hard. In the 1960s, Dr. Kilmer McCully not only warned that high levels of a particular amino acid called homocysteine could trigger heart attacks but suggested the simple remedy—the taking of folic acid in abundance, and foods containing the B vitamins. He was removed from his position and denied tenure, and his investigations were branded as unimportant. Since that time it is estimated about one-and-a-half million Americans have died of vascular disease related to homocysteine. I have read that the levels of homocysteine considered normal in McCully's time were actually responsible for tripling the incidence of heart disease. But neither the American Heart Association, nor the FDA, over the years between McCully's time and their own, have been wholehearted in promoting the only known remedy against the homocysteine danger—folic acid.

"What God has joined together, let no man put asunder." While originally said by Christ with reference to marriage, the principle applies to many things. In the Christian gospel, justification and sanctification are linked together, though the former takes precedence as the only way of producing the latter. Believers are saved by faith alone, but the faith that saves is never alone. There are many things that must be distinguished but never separated, such as members of the Trinity, or husband and wife. Similarly when God made food for man he knew exactly what he was doing for our health and happiness.

In 1900, we knew only rare cases of heart disease, because only carbohydrates were refined. There were no such things as trans fats. Most of the processed foods that now meet our eyes in the supermarket, in the packets, the cans, the bottles, lack many of the elements in the foods originally created by our Maker. The epidemics of heart disease and diabetes have taken place since we learned to process and refine foods. It is no coincidence that statistics about these two diseases run closely parallel. Wherever one is prominent in a culture, the other is there too, and in similar amounts. Both have been largely triggered by our refining and processing of foods, though a minority of sufferers may have genetic problems that have paved the way.

Approximately 9 percent of adult Americans have diabetes, and about one-third of Americans have some degree of insulin resistance which paves the way for diabetes. Before many years have passed, one in five on this continent will be diabetic.

In 1999, in the *Annals of Internal Medicine*, 130:89-96, you can read the article, "The Association Between Cardiorespiratory Fitness and Impaired Fasting Glucose and Type 2 Diabetes Mellitus in Men." The authors, W. M. Gibbon and L.W. Mitchell, record the study of nearly 9,000 men over 30 years of age whose health was tracked over six years. Over that period, 149 men developed diabetes, and these were almost always the most sedentary in the original group. The study showed that sedentary individuals were nearly four times as likely to develop diabetes, compared with physically active people.

All attempts to lose weight by diet alone yield only temporary success. Only when the correct diet is linked with regular physical activity can there be enduring change in weight.

Also, in 1999, *The American Journal of Epidemiology*, vol. 149:654-64, presented the article "Aging Successfully until Death in Old Age: Opportunities for Increasing Active Life Expectancy." The authors were S. G. Leveille and J. M. Gurilnik, and others. This article offers abundant evidence that people who regularly exercise are much less likely to become disabled than those who are sedentary. Very few men and women reaching the age of 80 are free of disability, but those who are physically active have greatly increased the likelihood of reaching this goal.

You are never too old to exercise, but newcomers to the habit should begin slowly and work up gradually. Numerous experiments have shown that people in their 80s and 90s, while increasing their activity, can drastically improve their muscle strength and their walking speed and coordination. Just walking dramatically reduces your likelihood of a heart attack and improves mental acuity. No special equipment or special training is needed. Put on a pair of sneakers and go. Increase your speed, as you are able.

Amid the flurry and confusion of conflicting opinions, remember that the key factors of diabetic therapy are diet and exercise. Some researchers go so far as to say that pills and insulin are for "lazy" diabetics who will not make the effort to control their disease by disciplined eating and physical activity. This is not always the case, but all those who discover they have diabetes type 2 should consider the criticism. For type 1 sufferers, of course, there is no alternative to insulin.

Strive to eat slowly, and thereby delay the rise in blood sugar. A meal that is well chatted over is not only a well-digested meal, but also one that is beneficial for the diabetic struggling to control his glucose figures.

Some diabetics have found the addition of vinegar or lemon juice to a meal slows the rise of blood sugar. Experiment and see if it works for you!

When it is dark enough, the eternal stars shine out bright enough. Discouragement is the anaesthetic the devil uses before he cuts out your heart. Remember Calvary and know that you are as greatly loved, as though there was nobody else to love. "If God be for us, who [or what] be against us?" God has a thousand ways of providing for us of which we know nothing. In every difficulty he has a way prepared to bring relief. "God has not given us the spirit of fear, but of power, and of love, and of a sound mind." (2 Tim 1:7)

APPENDIX B

Valuable Quotations for Diabetics Making Life-Style Changes

Here are some important insights by researchers to help guide the individual diabetic in making decisions. They cast light on the counsel, offered by most health-care teams, cognizant of recent studies about the use of monounsaturates in preference to carbohydrate intake.

The first source given, *Textbook on Diabetes*, edited by Pickup and Williams is the only one I would endorse without qualification. References takes from other volumes are not intended to endorse all the key positions set forth in those same books. *The Textbook on Diabetes* is a two-volume set running into hundreds of pages. It is a gold mine for those wishing to dig deeply into the treasure of tested and tried scientific diabetic lore.

> An epidemic of non-insulin dependent diabetes is occurring across the world...

> —edited by John C. Pickup and Garath Williams,
> *Textbook on Diabetes*, ch. 3, p. 17.

The NIDDM subjects will increase from 100 to 200 million worldwide in the next 15 years.

> —*Ibid.*

Diabetes mellitus is an important and rapidly growing problem in the developing world. The frequency of NIDDM is increasing rapidly in many developing countries, especially in urban populations. The advent of the Westernized life-style, with its excessive energy intake and reduced physical activity, is apparently responsible.

—Ibid., ch. 5, p. 1.

This same textbook says there's no botanical substitute for insulin, and though over 700 plants and herbs have been said to have sugar-reducing qualities, there's no scientific evidence of their adequacy. Even Guar gum, which slows down glucose rise, has not been proven to have significant value for overall glucose control. See chapters 5 and 84 of this textbook.

Diabetes mellitus is associated with over 50 worldwide genetic syndromes.

—Ibid., 28, p. 1.

The energy-dense, now Westernized diet, rich in fats and relatively low in carbohydrate and fiber in a setting of low physical activity, is a major cause of obesity and contributes to non-insulin dependent diabetes.

—Ibid., ch. 37, p. 1.

An acute reduction in energy intake reduces glycemia and may alleviate diabetic symptoms, even before significant weight loss occurs, but significant weight loss may be required to achieve significant glycemic metabolic control.

—Ibid.

An isocaloric diet rich in monounsaturated acids and low in saturated fats may provide a useful alternative to a high-carbohydrate diet for some people with NIDDM. Insulin insensitivity and dyslipidemia may all improve.

—Ibid.

Many patients find it difficult to persevere with high-carbohydrate, low-fat diets...a more palatable diet may be one that's enriched by monounsaturates (olive oil, grape seed oil) to replace saturated fats, rather than being severely restricted in fat content).

—Ibid., ch. 37, p. 7.

Now the MUFA rich diets may improve glycemic control, apparently by improving peripheral insensitivity. Moreover, plasma triglycerides and some-times HDL improve, while daytime blood pressure may also be reduced. MUFA's are also more resistant to lipid peroxidation than polyunsaturated fatty acids, and may contribute less to the pathogenesis of atherosclerosis. Short-term studies have shown that weight gain does not occur with isoca-loric MUFA diet.

—Ibid.

[This textbook quotes journal articles supporting the position taken.]

Exercise has acute and long-term effects, which are potentially beneficial for diabetic patients.

Exercise and physical training confer metabolic benefits in NIDDM, notably improved insulin sensitivity, enhanced glucose disposal, and a less athero-genic lipid profile with decreased plasma triglycerides and LDL.

—Ibid., ch. 37, p. 14.

Dietary modification remains the key to the treatment of NIDDM.

—*Ibid.*, ch. 37, p. 15.

Clinical and epidemiological data in humans suggest that the magnitude and duration of hyperglycemia are strongly associated with the severity of microvascular neuropathic complications.

—*Ibid.*, ch. 41, p. 1.

In the U.S., NIDDM accounts for more than 93 percent of cases of diabetes, and in the future will account almost certainly for a still larger proportion.

—*Ibid.*, ch. 41, p. 6.

Natural history of microvascular neuropathic complications of NIDDM has been difficult to define, for the disease may have been present for many years before it is diagnosed, and the incidence and progression of complications may be influenced by multiple confounding factors including age, hypertension, etc.

—*Ibid.*

Diet has long been suspected to play a part in diabetes. As early as the sixth century, Indian physicians attributed diabetes to a diet of over-rich foods, and by 1875 Bouchard had clearly described what we now call non-insulin dependent diabetes as being associated with obesity. He had also noted that rates of diabetes had declined during the siege of Paris. He attributed this to the food shortage of the time. Subsequently, Hindsworth showed that during the 1914-18 war, mortality rates declined markedly in Berlin and Paris—cities with serious food shortages—and to some extent London, whereas rates in New York and Tokyo remained constant or even possibly increased. Changes were also described in Europe during World War 1 and 2, and Japan in World War 2.

—Editors: Guido Bozza, Biero Micossi, Aldicol Cadabno, Rodolfo Baoletti, *Diet, Diabetes, and Atherosclerosis*, p. 109.

Obesity has been demonstrated to be a strong risk factor in the development of diabetes in several populations. In addition, the degree of genetic susceptibility for non-insulin diabetes is an extremely strong risk factor, as indicated by the rates of concordance in identical twins, and by the demonstration in populations that obesity and parental diabetes have synergistic effects upon the incidence of the disease. These two factors confound the interpretations of comparisons of diet in relation to diabetes. While food consumption among populations is also related to the incidence of diabetes, West was unable to find any evidence that calorie intake, or individual components of diet, independent of obesity, were implicated in its pathogenesis.

—*Ibid.*, p. 111.

Very low prevalences of diabetes have been noted among populations as diverse as Alaskan Eskimos, who consume relatively high-fat diets, the Broayas of the Sahara Desert, and the natives of the highlands of New Guinea who consume predominately complex carbohydrates. The number of other populations which have undergone rapid change in their way of life, including Yemenite Jews immigrating to Israel, Australian Aborigines moving to an urban environment, and many Pacific populations show unusually high prevalence of diabetes. Very high prevalence of diabetes, for example, has been found in the republic of Nauru, a country which emerged from being a typical Pacific island community with reliance on fishing and local food, and has become the richest country in the world in terms of per capita income. Here the prevalence of diabetes among those 20 years of age and older is now over 30 percent, and obesity is rampant. In other Pacific islands, there are striking differences in the rates of diabetes in islanders still living in their traditional environment, and those who have moved to an urban environment; yet in such migrant populations the genetic susceptibility to diabetes is exactly the same as those who have moved to the urban environment and now consume diets very different to their traditional food. There are several diseases associated with such change. Obesity, hypertension, dental caries, coronary disease, and hyperuricemia, and gout, as well as diabetes appear to increase in frequency. Typically in such communities the diet changes from one characterized by the consumption of local fruit and vegetables (usually with a high fiber and carbohydrate content) supplemented by fish, to one characterized by the consumption of large quantities of rice, flour, and sugar. Consumption of calories primarily from refined carbohydrates increases considerably, whereas the consumption of traditional vegetables such as taro, yams, which are high in complex carbohydrates and fiber decreases. For example, the dietary intake in Nauruans is now estimated to be over 7,000 calories in males and over 5,000 in females. The amount of fruit consumed typically decreases, whereas the amount of sugar increases, along with salt intake and saturated fat consumption. At the same time, levels of physical activity decrease.

—Ibid., p. 112.

Another unusual population with calorie intake in the range of 4,500-6,400 calories a day is the Sumo wrestlers of Japan. In contrast, the typical Japanese diet consists of about 2,400 calories. Most of the Sumo are more than 50 percent overweight and consume about 80 percent of their total calories as carbohydrates. The Sumo are recruited as adolescents, and undergo a period of training for about seven years before entering an active wrestling period which usually lasts about ten years. They must be sufficiently obese and heavy to be effective competitors in the ring. Of 158 wrestlers between 15 and 31 years of age, 18 percent were found to have glucose intolerance, and diabetes is reported to be extremely common (more than 40 percent) in retired wrestlers.

—Ibid.

Like other Pacific islanders, the prevalence of diabetes in Japanese who migrated to the Pacific islands is higher than in their own homeland. Careful comparison of prevalence of diabetes and diet has been made among Japanese subjects residing in Hiroshima and in the island of Hawaii. In Hawaii the prevalence of diabetes is approximately twice that of the same age groups in Hiroshima, and obesity is approximately seven times as frequent. In spite of the difference and prevalence of diabetes and obesity, the number of calories consumed by Hawaiian Japanese was not different to that of the inhabitants of Hiroshima. Hawaiian Japanese, however, consume twice as much fat, one third less complex carbohydrate, almost three times as much simple carbohydrate, as their counterparts in Hiroshima. The frequency of heart disease is also higher in Hawaii than in Hiroshima...And the level of physical activity frequently changes.

—Ibid., p. 114.

Another prospective study is among the Pima Indians of Arizona. The Pima Indians have the highest known prevalence and incidents of diabetes in the world. The prevalence reaches roughly 50 percent in persons age 35 and over.

—Ibid.

Diabetics not only face shortened life spans but also suffer significant diabetes-related complications. Each year...more than 55,000 lower extremity complications or amputations take place, 13,300 of end stage renal disease, and 15,000 new cases of blindness. There are also annually 2.7 million hospitalizations for diabetes and 3.3 million persons with long-term reduction in physical activity.

—published by the U.S. Department of Health, *Diabetes in US: Strategy for Prevention,* Foreword.

Diabetes is a global health problem. A 1994 Study estimated that approximately 100 million people around the world have diabetes, and that by the year 2010, the number would rise to more than 215 million. These estimates were made before the current, more inclusive definition of diabetes was accepted in 1997. Under the new definition, prevalence of diabetes in the world was more like 140 million in 1994 and will be 300 million in 2010.

Diabetes is concentrated where food supplies allow people to eat more calories than they need, so that they develop obesity, a condition of excessive fat. There are actually several different types of diabetes, but the type usually associated with obesity, called type 2 diabetes (see Chapter 3), far outweighs the other types.

—Alan L. Rubin, M.D., *Diabetes for Dummies*, p. 22.

Large-scale studies have shown that the average hemoglobin A1c in the United States for type 2 diabetes is around 9.4 percent, which means the average blood glucose is 220. The American Diabetes Association recommends taking action to control the blood glucose if the hemoglobin A1c is 8 percent or greater, with the goal being less than 7 percent.

—*Ibid.*

Controlling the blood pressure is absolutely essential in diabetes. The goal in diabetes is an even lower blood pressure than in the nondiabetic, because studies have shown that lower normal blood pressures result in less diabetic damage than higher normal blood pressures. Blood pressure should be no higher than 130/85, and 120/80 is even better.

How well are doctors doing at controlling blood pressure in people with diabetes? A study has shown that only 15 percent of people with diabetes with hypertension have a blood pressure as low as 140/90, and only 5 percent have a blood pressure down to 130/85.

—*Ibid.*, p. 120.

If there were a more controversial area in nutrition for the diabetic person than carbohydrates, I would like to know about it. For years, the American Diabetes Association told people with diabetes that they should be eating 55 to 60 percent of their calories as carbohydrate. Other experts said that that amount was too much. Some even said that that amount was too little. The ADA has now modified its recommendation so that it says in the Clinical Practice Recommendations for 1998: "The percent of carbohydrate will vary and is individualized based on the individual's eating habits and glucose and lipid (fat) goals." In this section, I give you my suggestion for carbohydrate in your diet based on my reading of the medical literature and my clinical experience. You are free to disagree with me and use whatever level of carbohydrate you like, as long as it helps to promote a lower blood glucose, without increasing blood fats or weight.

—Ibid., p. 125.

Although the fat intake of the American population has declined because of the fear of coronary artery disease caused by cholesterol, Americans are getting fatter. In fact, 55 percent of Americans are considered overweight or obese. Because Americans are not eating more protein, the culprit is most probably excess carbohydrate, such as that found in concentrated sweets like pastry and candy as well as the more complex carbohydrate found in bread. Within the body, carbohydrate can be turned into fat and stored. This function was great when everyone lived in caves and got little food for prolonged periods of time, but it doesn't fit today's life-style, consisting as it does of abundant food (and minimal foraging for it in the supermarket).

Because carbohydrate is the food that raises the blood glucose, which is responsible for the complications of diabetes, it seems right to recommend a diet that is lower in carbohydrate than previously suggested. Furthermore, a major source of coronary artery disease in diabetes is the insulin resistance syndrome (see Chapter 5). Because increased carbohydrate triggers increased triglycerides, which is the beginning of a number of abnormalities that lead to increased coronary artery disease, recommending less carbohydrate on this basis as well seems prudent.

My experience has been that a diet of 40 percent carbohydrate makes controlling my patients' blood glucose much easier.

—Ibid., p. 126.

Monounsaturated fats do not raise cholesterol. Avocado, olive oil, and canola oil are examples. The oil in nuts like almonds and peanuts is monounsaturated.

—Ibid., p. 131.

Your diet must contain sufficient vitamins and minerals, but the amount you need may be less than you think. If you eat a balanced diet than comes from the various food groups, you generally get enough vitamins for your daily needs.

—Ibid., p. 132.

No scientific evidence shows that chromium is especially helpful to the person with diabetes in controlling the blood glucose despite reams of articles in health food magazines to the contrary.

—Ibid., p. 134.

In making a choice among the first-generation drugs, tolbutamide, acetohex-amide, and tolazamide are considered less potent, and chlorpropamide is felt to be the most potent of them. If the first three (of which tolbutamide is the mildest) do not work, then chlorpropamide is tried. If chlorpropamide doesn't lower the blood glucose sufficiently, then the second-generation drugs are used. Doctors, too often, do not try the first-generation drugs today and go right to the second-generation pills. For many people, the second-generation pills are too potent, and hypoglycemia becomes a problem. For others, the second-generation drugs provide no greater benefit than the earlier ones. All these drugs suffer from the fact that, sooner or later, they no longer control the blood glucose.

—Ibid., p. 159.

...troglitazone does have some problems:

- It may cause liver damage, and some early deaths were associated with its use before this was understood. The current recommendation is that a liver test be done before and monthly for the first 12 months after starting treatment and then quarterly thereafter. If the specific liver tests called ALT rise more than three times the upper limit of normal, the drug must be stopped. Once it is stopped, the liver abnormality almost always disappears.

- It causes water retention and swelling of the ankles, especially in the older population, which some people do not find tolerable. Occasionally, the drug is stopped for this reason.

- It should not be taken by a pregnant woman with diabetes or a nursing mother.

—Ibid., p. 163.

Repaglinide, brand name Prandin, is the last of the current group of new medications for type 2 diabetes. It's the first of a group of drugs called *meglitinides*, which are chemically unrelated to the sulfonylureas but work by squeezing more insulin out of the pancreas just like the sulfonylureas do. Repaglinide, however, is taken just before meals to stimulate insulin for only that meal.

—Ibid., p. 164.

The effect of increased carbohydrate intake on insulin stimulation has been disastrous. We now know that obese patients and most people with type 2 diabetes have elevated blood insulin levels, which contribute to further weight gain.

—Calvin Ezrin, M.D. & Robert E. Kowalski, *The Type 2 Diabetes Diet Book*, p. XIV.

The link between obesity and high blood pressure has long been noted in medicine. Now we know that this is owing to insulin resistance; there is a high prevalence of hypertension in insulin-resistant individuals. Indeed, one can actually measure the influence of weight on blood pressure. For every kilogram of weight gained over one's healthy weight (that's 2.2 pounds), blood pressure goes up to .2 to .3 mm/Hg (millimeters of mercury on the doctor's blood pressure meter).

—Ibid., p. 12.

Commonly prescribed high-carbohydrate diets produce higher plasma glucose and insulin levels.

—Ibid., p. 13.

…Such diets generate significantly higher triglycerides and lower HDL levels…

—Ibid., p. 13.

A diet low in carbohydrates prevents those adverse responses. On this program, blood sugar and insulin levels fall dramatically, as does the level of triglycerides.

—Ibid., p. 13.

At the 1996 meeting of the American Diabetic Association, researchers agreed that while various medications are helpful, "Our studies show that low-intensity, prolonged exercise—such as a daily brisk walk of forty-five minutes to an hour—will substantially reduce insulin levels, thus reducing the risk of both diabetes and heart disease," said Dr. Jean-Pierre Despres of Laval University Hospital in Quebec.

—Ibid., p. 15.

Canadian researchers in 1996 reported in the *New England Journal of Medicine* that high fasting insulin concentrations in the blood appear to be an independent predictor of coronary artery disease. That is to say, even if cholesterol and blood pressure are controlled, and one stops smoking, hyperinsulinemia remains a factor increasing the risk of heart disease. How? The body's inability to use insulin for glucose metabolism is strongly related to atherosclerosis, the blockage in the coronary arteries, which supply the muscle of the heart with blood and oxygen.

—*Ibid.*, p. 16.

It's no coincidence that approximately 25 percent of the population has elevated levels of insulin in the blood and that about the same number of people—or perhaps more—are at least 20 percent overweight and sedentary. The answer for all is weight control and exercise.

—*Ibid.*, p. 17.

Dr. Atkins published his *Diet Revolution*. In it he advocated strict avoidance of carbohydrates, but allowed all the meat and fat one wanted to eat. Because the diet worked, and readers lost weight as promised, this approach became popular. But the diet had a number of flaws. Dieters' cholesterol levels rose significantly, increasing the risk of heart disease. The state of ketosis produced by the diet was uncontrolled. When readers returned to their former eating habits, they quickly regained the lost weight.

—*Ibid.*, p. 43.

Certainly insulin has its heroic side. But until recently the malevolent side of the hormone has been ignored. Ironically, the negative physiologic effects of insulin have been well documented. Insulin controls fat buildup and breakdown, as well as salt and water retention. It is the fat-building hormone generating triglycerides from carbohydrate precursors in the liver, and also in adipose tissue, where they are stored as energy reserves. Insulin also blocks fat breakdown via inhibition of the lipolytic action of growth hormone, glucagon, and catecholamines on the hormone-sensitive lipase in adipocytes.

Insulin is the second most powerful salt-retaining hormone, next to aldosterone. Without excessive intake of calories, it can produce rapid weight gain from fluid retention alone.

—*Ibid.*, p. 285.

There are four major causes for the development of insulin resistance. First is obesity itself, developed over time, in which adipose tissue produces a substance that moves to muscle tissue to selectively block the blood sugar-lowering effect of insulin. The second cause is type 2 diabetes, in which insulin resistance may precede diabetes and may or may not be associated with obesity. Third, when blood sugar levels exceed 300, or perhaps even less, the hyperglycemia can trigger insulin resistance. The fourth cause is stress, whether physical, emotional, or traumatic, that increases insulin-neutralizing stress hormones including cortisol, adrenaline, glucagon, and growth hormone.

—*Ibid.*, p. 285.

There are a number of myths surrounding diet and diabetes, and much of what is still considered sensible nutritional advice for diabetics can over the long run be fatal. I know, because it almost killed me. I developed diabetes in 1946 at the age of twelve, and for more than two decades I was an "ordinary" diabetic, dutifully following doctor's orders…

—*Dr. Bernstein's Diabetes Solution*, p. I.

Over the years, the complications from my diabetes became worse and worse, and like many diabetics in similar circumstances, I faced a very early death.

—*Ibid.*, p. i.

During my twenties and thirties, the prime of life for most people, many of my body's systems began to deteriorate. I had excruciatingly painful kidney stones, a stone in a salivary duct, "frozen" shoulders, a progressive deformity of my feet with impaired sensation…

—Ibid., p. xvi.

…My wife, a physician, pointed out to me that I had spent much of my life going into, experiencing, or recovering from hypoglycemia, which is a state of excessively low blood sugar. It was usually accompanied by fatigue and headaches. During these episodes, I became confused and unruly and snapped at people. The strain on my family was clearly becoming untenable.

—Ibid., p. xvii.

Within a year, I had refined my insulin and diet regimen to the point that I had essentially normal blood sugars around the clock. After years of chronic fatigue and debilitating complications, almost overnight I was no longer continually tired or "washed out." After years of sky-high readings, my serum cholesterol and triglyceride levels had now not only dropped, but were at the low end of the normal ranges.

—Ibid., pp. xix–xx.

…Every few months I'd read another article saying that blood sugar normalization wasn't even remotely possible. How was it that I, an engineer, had figured out how to do what was impossible for medical professionals? I was deeply grateful for the fortuitous combination of events that had turned my life, my health, and my family around and put me on the right path. At the very least, I felt, I was obliged to share my newfound knowledge with others.

There were no doubt millions of "ordinary" diabetics like me suffering needlessly.

—Ibid., p. xxi.

...By 1977 I was able to get the first of two university-sponsored studies started in the New York City area. These both succeeded in reversing early complications in diabetic patients. As a result of our successes, the two universities separately sponsored the world's first two symposia on blood glucose self-monitoring. By this time I was being invited to speak at international diabetes conferences, but rarely at meetings in the United States. Curiously, more physicians *outside* the United States seemed interested in controlling blood sugar than did their American colleagues.

—Ibid., p. xxii.

You're the only person who can be responsible for normalizing your blood sugar. Although your physician may guide you, the ultimate responsibility is in your hands. This task will require significant changes in life-style that may involve some sacrifice.

—Ibid., p. 3.

Perhaps the most curious fact about diet, nutrition, and medication is that while we can make accurate generalizations about how most of us will react to a particular diet or medical regimen, each individual will react somewhat differently to a given food.

—Ibid., p. 108.

...Many contemporary dietary researchers exploring this phenomenon have begun to arrive at the conclusion that a high-carbohydrate diet is not so benign. In fact, it has been shown—and it is my own observation—that such a diet can increase body weight, increase blood insulin levels, and raise most cardiac risk factors.

—Ibid., p. 110.

When I was on a very low-fat, high-carbohydrate diet thirty years ago, I had high triglycerides (usually over 250 mg/dl) and high serum cholesterol (usually over 300 mg/dl), and I developed a number of vascular complications. When I went on to a very low-carbohydrate diet and did not restrict my fat, the same thing happened to me that happened to Arctic explorer Stefansson, but more so—my lipids plummeted. Now, at sixty-three, I have the lipid profile of an Olympic athlete, apparently from eating a low-carbohydrate diet in order to normalize my blood sugars. That I exercise regularly probably doesn't hurt my lipid profile, either…

—Ibid., p. 115.

One purpose of blood glucose self-monitoring is to learn through your blood sugar profiles how particular foods affect you. Over years of examining these profiles, I've observed that some people are more tolerant of certain foods than other people. For example, bread makes my own blood sugar rise very rapidly. Yet some of my patients eat a sandwich of thin bread every day with only minor problems. This is inevitably related to delayed stomach-emptying (see Chapter 21). In any case, you should feel free to experiment with food and then perform blood sugar readings.

—Ibid., pp. 121-122.

Milk contains a considerable amount of the simple sugar lactose and will rapidly raise blood sugar. Skim milk actually contains more lactose per ounce than does whole milk. One or two teaspoons of milk in a cup of coffee will not significantly affect blood sugar, but 1/4 cup of milk will make a considerable difference to most of us.

—Ibid., p. 127.

Cottage cheese also contains a considerable amount of lactose because, unlike most other cheeses, which are okay, it is only partly fermented. I was unaware of this until several patients showed me records of substantial blood sugar increases after consuming a small container of cottage cheese. It should be avoided except in very small amounts, say about two tablespoons.

—Ibid., p. 127.

...In 1997, the Centers for Disease Control and Prevention (CDC) reported the number of Americans with diabetes had increased six-fold over the past forty years, and in 1998, the American Diabetes Association reported that the incidence of type 2 diabetes increased by 9 percent per year between 1987 and 1996.

—Janet Worsley Norwood & Charles B. Inlander,
Understanding Diabetes, p. 2.

When it was approved, experts heralded troglitazone as a development that would revolutionize the treatment of diabetes. Whether the drug is a breakthrough, however, remains to be seen. Only months after its approval, its manufacturer, Warner-Lambert, issued warnings to practitioners, advising them to watch carefully for liver problems in those on the drug. In December 1997, troglitazone was pulled from the market in England because of serious effects on the liver reported by patients in both the United States and Japan.

—Ibid., p. 92.

Primary failure happens when the drugs don't work in the first place. This happens about 20 to 30 percent of the time—a fairly substantial number.

Secondary failure happens when the drug quits working after it has been used successfully for a while.

—*Ibid.*, p. 95.

Secondary failure is a significant problem. Each year, there's a 5 to 10 percent chance that a person on oral therapy will experience secondary failure. The medical world hoped that the second-generation sulfonylureas would be less vulnerable to this problem, but that doesn't seem to be the case...

—*Ibid.*, p. 96.

Eventually, 60 to 70 percent of patients with type 2 diabetes who are being treated aggressively need insulin treatment.

—*Ibid.*, p. 98.

Quite simply, the longer you have diabetes, the greater your chance of developing retinopathy. Within ten years of diabetes diagnosis, half of all people with type 1 diabetes and a quarter with type 2 have some damage to their retinas. By twenty years after diagnosis of diabetes, nearly everyone with type 1 diabetes and over 60 percent with type 2 have some degree of retinopathy.

—*Ibid.*, p. 120.

Officially known as diabetic nephropathy, nephropathy is a type of kidney disease that leads to kidney failure. Nephropathy tends to develop in people who have had diabetes for 20 years or more. It used to be that a third of all people with type 1 diabetes developed nephropathy, but today's treatment methods and the emphasis on better blood-sugar control are shrinking that percentage. People with type 2 diabetes develop nephropathy infrequently.

—*Ibid.*, p. 127.

Cardiovascular disease is the most common complication of type 2 diabetes. In fact, people with diabetes have a risk of cardiovascular disease that is two to five times that of people without the condition.

—*Ibid.*, p. 129.

Heart attacks and strokes are more common in people with type 2 diabetes than in those with type 1 diabetes, yet medical science is not sure exactly why this is. Experts believe it could be because people with type 2 diabetes tend to be overweight. (Obesity is a known risk factor for heart attack and stroke.)

—*Ibid.*, p. 130.

Triglycerides (sometimes known as **VLDL**, or very-low-density lipoprotein) are another form of fat in the body. High levels of triglycerides in the blood (**hypertriglyceridemia**) may not directly cause arteriosclerosis but may accompany other abnormalities that speed its development. People with diabetes tend to have high levels of triglycerides, too. Combine high triglyceride levels of 200 to 500 mg/dL with cholesterol levels between 200 and 300 mg/dL, and you have what *The American Heart Journal* calls *combined* **hyperlipidemia**, meaning too much fat. Triglycerides more than 500 mg/dl and/or cholesterol levels over 300 mg/dL are called massive hyperlipidemia. Combined and *massive hyperlipidemia* are found in over 30 percent of all people with diabetes—approximately two to three times more often than in people without diabetes.

—*Ibid.*, p. 132.

More than half of all lower-limb amputations in the United States are performed on people with diabetes. Each year, reports the American Podiatric Medical Association, the number of lower-limb amputations due to diabetic complications in the United States exceeds the number of limbs lost worldwide to land mines. Almost half of these 67,000 amputations could have been prevented through early detection and treatment.

—Ibid, p. 138.

Recognizing Risk Factors

As is true with all diabetic complications, certain factors increase risk of foot problems. The greatest of these is smoking. According to the American Diabetes Association, of the people with diabetes who need amputations, almost all are smokers.

—*Ibid.*, p. 138.

Unlike many other illnesses, *most of the control of diabetes rests in the hands of the patient.* Self-care is not just important, it's absolutely essential.

—*Ibid.*, p. 141.

Managing your diabetes is demanding and, at times, difficult. It's a daily, lifelong process. And even when you try your best, your condition can still get out of hand. But the alternative—neglecting the disease—poses such demonstrated drawbacks that most folks opt for self-care.

—*Ibid.*, p. 142.

Researchers think that large amounts of carbohydrates increase triglyceride levels in poorly controlled type 2 diabetes.

Another diet, this one low in carbohydrates, has been devised by Richard K. Bernstein, M.D., in his book *Diabetes Type 2* (New York: Prentice Hall, 1990). He recommends that people with type 2 diabetes eat only 30 grams of carbohydrates a day—equivalent to 2 slices of bread.

Bernstein argues that a high-carbohydrate meal makes it impossible to attain normal blood-sugar levels for several hours after eating, and he strives to keep blood-sugar levels normal at all points in the day. (In contrast, most doctors expect and accept a higher postprandial, or after-meal, blood-sugar reading.)

—Ibid., p. 158.

If you have type 2 diabetes and have difficulty digesting high-fiber carbohy-drates, or if a high-fiber, high-carbohydrate diet doesn't seem to control your blood sugar, then you might wish to consider a low-carbohydrate diet.

—Ibid., p. 159.

Very large amounts of caffeine (five to ten cups of coffee a day) may raise blood sugar. Furthermore, the adverse effects of too much caffeine are often confused with signs of an insulin reaction, or vice versa: anxiety, trembling, and irritability.

—Ibid., p. 172.

Excessive drinking, however, is likely to wreak havoc with a blood-glucose level, sending it spiraling downward by interfering with the way the liver processes glycogen.

In addition, diabetic drugs known as oral hypoglycemic agents (especially first-generation oral agents—see Chapter 3) may interact with alcohol, caus-ing facial flushing, severe headaches, or dizziness.

—Ibid., p. 172.

...A carefully planned vegetarian diet can be very healthy. Long-term retro-spective studies of vegetarians find that they live longer and healthier lives than their peers who eat the typical American high-protein, high-fat diet.

—Ibid., p. 175.

The American Diabetes Association, for its part, does not recommend any herb for treating diabetes because there is no scientific evidence herbs are helpful. In fact, in some instances they may be harmful. For example, certain herbs may interact poorly with diabetes medications.

—Ibid., p. 176.

People with diabetes must begin exercise programs as early in the course of their disease as possible, before it's too late to reap exercise's many benefits.

—Ibid., p. 181.

…The biggest reason to give up smoking is that it increases the risk of diabetic complications such as cardiovascular and kidney disease by accelerating small-blood-vessel damage. Recent research also shows that the sugars in tobacco—which enter the body through cigarette smoke—undergo chemical reactions in the body, ultimately forming clumps of cholesterol and other substances that stick to and clog artery walls. People with diabetes already have higher rates of cardiovascular and kidney complication—why compound the risk?

—Ibid., p. 184.

Physicians, diabetes-teaching nurses, and dieticians usually advocate one type of diet—usually the one they were initially taught in their training and have recommended to their patients ever since. They often become disturbed and even angry at the suggestion that there may be a different, possibly even better, diet for people with diabetes.

—Peter A. Lodewick, M.D., June Biermann, and Barbara Toohey,
The Diabetic Man, p. 188.

...The majority of patients, when they first come to see me are on the middle-ground diet. They have the idea that a healthy diet is high in complex carbohydrates. They have had it grilled into them every day that having fat in the diet and eating eggs is hostile to blood cholesterol and the cause of vascular disease. However, most of my patients don't stay on this middle-ground diet. Usually the reason that they come to see me is because they can't get good diabetes control, are overweight, and run high cholesterol and triglycerides on the diet they are following.

—Ibid., p. 119.

...Sometimes cutting back on carbohydrates early on will rapidly improve high blood sugars.

—Ibid., p. 119.

My experience with the low-carbohydrate diet has been for the most part extremely good. Your irate dietitian friend who was concerned about promoting kidney failure among people with diabetes is way out of line.

—Ibid., p. 122.

When people convert from a high-calorie diet with plenty of carbohydrates to a low-carbohydrate diet, the amount of protein they consume is not that much greater anyway. The improved blood sugars that result from a lower-carbohydrate diet far offset any potential damage that a very high-protein diet may bring about.

—Ibid., p. 122.

Dr. Julian Whitaker, who in most of his books (for example, *Reversing Diabetes*) espoused the high carbohydrate diet, recently said in his Health and Healing Newsletter, "When, with good reason, it becomes necessary for one to separate from a dogma that one has long supported, it's best to go ahead, do it, and get it over with. For years I have advocated a diet very high in complex carbohydrates. While I maintain my stance on the deleterious effects of excessive fats, new research has convinced me that excessive carbohydrates pose similar risks."

—Ibid., p. 123.

Alcohol is a toxic substance that has many deleterious effects on your body and mind. These effects can include muscle aches, sleeplessness, anxiety, depression, diminished sex drive, increased cholesterol and triglycerides, liver damage, greater susceptibility to cataracts, osteoporosis (even in men), and gastrointestinal disorders. Heavy drinking does some of its most serious damage to your nervous system, where it causes neuritis and neuropathy.

—Ibid., p. 144.

At a recent annual meeting of the American Diabetes Association, they emphasized that diabetics consuming two to four ounces of alcohol per day have a much higher incidence of neuropathy than those who don't drink.

—Ibid., p. 144.

If the acute effects of alcohol intoxication and/or associated hypoglycemia don't cause a catastrophe for your diabetes control, then a wicked hangover looms over you like a great buzzard. The dizziness, vertigo, nausea, vomiting, and headache of a horrible hangover can be so severe that they will wreak havoc with your diabetes. The stress of such a tumultuous condition can raise the blood sugar.

—Ibid., p. 147.

As is the case with any drug, metformin does have some side effects. Metformin is contraindicated, that is, should not be prescribed, in patients with heart, kidney, or liver disease. Approximately 20 percent of patients taking metformin complain of gastrointestinal distress after taking the drug. These gastrointestinal problems range from a bitter metallic aftertaste in the mouth to diarrhea. It has been found that these unpleasant side effects tend to diminish after some time on the drug.

From 1959 to 1977, doctors prescribed phenformin (trade named Meltrol, a close relative of metformin) to hundreds of thousands of type 2 diabetics. In 1977 the FDA identified over two hundred cases of lactic acidosis in patients who were using this drug and banned the use of phenformin in this country.

—Joseph Juliano, M.D., *The Diabetic Male's Essential Guide to Living Well*, pp. 17-18.

If you feel a little intimidated over the lancet and drop of blood, do not let it bother you one bit. Just know that many others have felt and do feel exactly the same way. And remember also; do not sweat the small stuff. The tremendous benefits you will derive from better control of your diabetes far outweigh the minor inconvenience of checking your blood sugar regularly.

—*Ibid.*, p. 24.

"People deny reality. They fight against real feelings caused by real circumstances. They build mental worlds of shoulds, oughts, and might have beens. Real changes only begin with real appraisal and acceptance of what is. Only then is realistic action possible." These are the worlds of David Reynolds, an American exponent of Japanese Morita Psychotherapy, about personal behavior.

—*Ibid.*, p. 50.

Renal insufficiency, or kidney disease and failure, is the largest cause of death in the diabetic population in those who are diagnosed with this disease before age twenty.

—*Ibid.*, p. 62.

After fifteen years of diabetes, approximately 33 percent of those with type 1 diabetes and 20 percent of those with type 2 diabetes will develop diabetic nephropathy. Factors associated with a higher incidence of diabetic nephropathy within the diabetic population are hypertension, poor blood sugar control, and smoking.

Fortunately, today we have several defenses to fight against these factors.

—*Ibid.*, pp. 62-63.

Ever since statistics have been kept for this disease, the incidence and prevalence rates of ESRD [end-stage renal disease] treatments have increased without showing signs of letting up. The age-, race-, and gender-adjusted incidence rate of ESRD treatment increased by 7.8 percent per year between 1985-1987 and 1988-1990. By 1990, the number of patients treated for ESRD amounted to two hundred ten thousand annually. Current projections predict the number may be close to three hundred thousand by the year 2000.

Diabetes may account for up to 33 percent of all cases of ESRD in the United States. The risk of ESRD is much greater with type 1 diabetes than type 2. Although there is a greater preponderance of type 2 diabetes, about 80 percent of the fourteen to fifteen million diagnosed cases of diabetes, type 1 diabetes still accounts for about 66 percents of all causes of diabetic ESRD.

—*Ibid.*, p. 67.

Capsaicin, an extract from hot peppers that gives them their fiery taste, is a new hope for diabetics who experience painful peripheral neuropathy. This drug is found naturally in the peppers that are used to make Tabasco sauce and some salsas, a traditional dish of spices, peppers, and other ingredients often combined in a tomato base. I eat a lot of salsa and I find that the natural capsaicin in the peppers has reduced my neuropathy to zero. I have not suffered any neuropathy pain in years, and salsa is always part of my lunch. Capsaicin can now be purchased at health-food stores and pharmacies. Ask your doctor; there should be no problem in taking it to help prevent neuropathy because this is a safe, naturally occurring product.

Some of the older physicians who treat long-term diabetics have reported that vitamin B12 injections (sometimes in conjunction with thiamine) have alleviated some painful diabetic neuropathy.

—Ibid., pp. 71.

Some of you may think that the term **positive attitudinal healing** sounds pretty fancy or that it is strictly a bunch of bunk, or you may already know a lot about it. I refer you to *The Healing Brain*, edited by Robert Ornstein and Charles Swencionis, which details the scientific studies that have revealed evidence of the various psychological states and life traumas that can adversely affect the immune system. There is much scientific evidence in support of this theory. Eminent psychiatrists, psychologists, and neuroscientists describe investigations into the mind-brain-body relationships that are changing our understanding of the illness process. It is fascinating reading.

—Ibid., p. 88.

Over the last several years, it had been thought that increasing carbohydrate intake was okay for the diabetic, and that diabetics as well as marathon runners and those engaging in extreme sports could benefit from a diet rich in complex carbohydrates, including large amounts of pasta, beans, potatoes, and rice. However, the newest findings indicate that this intake leads to higher blood glucose values and weight gain, so it is now recommended that the diabetic carefully monitor the amount of simple and complex carbohydrates consumed.

—*Ibid.*, p. 110.

The incidence of diabetes seems to be quite high all over the world but in some areas, such as rural Africa, the incidence is low. Why is this? Where there is a large dietary intake of unrefined foods, fruits, and vegetables, and an almost total lack of fat, sugar, and meat, there is very little, if any, diabetes. As scientists began studying eating behavior, it was seen again and again that in areas of high dietary fiber intake, the incidence of diabetes was low. In areas where there was little dietary fiber intake, the incidence of diabetes was high. It has become alarmingly evident that Americans do not include enough fiber in their diets. During the last three decades, through commercial processing, we have lost fiber in some of our most often consumed foods, such as the husks of grains and rice and the skins of fruits and vegetables.

—*Ibid.*, p. 117.

Diabetes is a full-time challenge and will not ever give you a break, especially when you feel you need it the most. A special kind of stamina is required to live with this incurable disease for a lifetime, and special mental conditioning will certainly assist you. Your adherence to meticulous discipline and the necessary care your diabetes requires will also assist in getting you through the difficult times.

—*Ibid.*, p. 172.

Recent studies indicate that a diet high in monounsaturated fat and low in carbohydrate can produce a more desirable plasma glucose, lipid, and insulin profile in the short term. Others have shown beneficial effects from a monounsaturated fat diet compared with a high carbohydrate diet of one or both glycaemic control and lipids, without leading to weight gain despite the diet being higher in fat. Others have reported weight loss in the caloric restricted diet that are higher. Monounsaturated diet resulted in better gly-caemic control as well as weight loss in patients with NIDDM.

In the presence of elevated tryglicerides, increased monounsaturated fats (20% of total) are recommended leaving 50% of the remaining caloric intake to carbohydrates.

—Dr. Sophia Cauzos, Ms. Sue Metcalf, Dr. Richard Murray, Dr. Sharon O'Rourke. *Systematic Review of Existing Evidence and Primary Care Guidelines on the Management of Non Insulin Dependent Diabetes in Aboriginal and Torres Strait Islander Populations*, Kimberley Aboriginal Medical Services Council. The Office for Aboriginal and Torres Strait Island Health Services, Commonwealth Department of Health and Family Services, Canberra ACT, 1997, pp. 59, 60.

APPENDIX C

Handling Stress

It is absolutely vital to understand that experience is not what happens to us but what we do with what happens to us. And what we do with what happens to us depends upon our own hearts and minds. The relationship between mind and body is very intimate. Each affects the other tremendously. When the Bible declares that, as we think, so we are, it is setting forth not only a psychological truth but also a physiological one. Think of how we shed tears when the mind is burdened with sorrows. Think of the way in which we sweat when we are scared and fearful, and how the temperature of the hands and feet can change. Remember the white face of someone who suddenly received a fright. Remember your own racing heart when excited, and the pant of passion, and the sob of horror. All of these things are the physiological results of thinking.

The mind initiates all such changes. When something upsets us or puts us on tension the hypothalamus behind the cerebrum is greatly stirred and it influences the pituitary, the master of all the endocrine glands, particularly the adrenals. And the hormones from these glands secreted into the blood affect every cell of the body. This is why sometimes we can't sleep at night if something exciting or stressful or worrying has come up just before bedtime. The adrenals have sent adrenaline through the body and mind. The adrenaline is there in case we have to fight or take flight. When we do neither, but go to bed, we do not lose consciousness until the adrenaline has drained away from each cell of the brain.

It would be worth a million dollars to each of us just to remember this simple fact—feelings follow thoughts. When we choose our regular thoughts, we choose our regular feelings. All depression that is not hormonal or chemical springs from wrong thinking. We cannot indulge bitterness or anger or anxiety without precipitating feelings of depression.

Observe how very practical these matters are. If our mind triggers our bodies, and if our thoughts trigger our feelings, then there are obviously golden rules to obey if we wish to avoid being overcome by the stresses of life. We shall no more permit negative thoughts to reign in our minds than we would permit a burglar to set up house in our home.

Roger Babson, the great statistician, was once asked, "How come you have lived so long and so well?" He said, "We have a rule in our house, that we don't say anything negative after sundown." That's a mighty good rule. It also applies at all mealtimes. We should never discuss things that cause wrong thoughts, negative thoughts, at mealtime. Never eat when you're sad, mad, or bad. Some might die of starvation if they take me too literally, but the principle remains true.

We are not what we think we are, but what we think, we are. For example, a man's own view of himself and his conclusion to the issue of whether life has meaning will greatly determine the intensity of his personal stresses. If he sees himself as of no value, and feels he deserves troubles, then his self-worthlessness increases. Every sorrow that comes his way he will take as a judgment and a punishment and his self-worth will be diminished still further. He finds it impossible to be "loyal to the royal in himself." In contrast, the person who has found the gospel, who knows that God gave his Son for sinners and welcomes them—that person can handle stress as one who already has the richest yields of existence in his grasp. Such persons will remember that the north wind made the Vikings and that kites rise high against the wind. In other words they will view the stresses and strains of life as part of divine discipline to help them mature and grow.

Remember the wild Helen Keller? From two years of age, she was blind, deaf, and violent. She was violent because she was angry, and she was angry because she couldn't make sense of life. But Ann Sullivan taught her that everything has a name and that everything is loved. One day Ann had tried to spell out the word "water" to Helen, but Helen could not understand the message. In her anger she tore her doll to shreds and tramped out of the house. Ann went before her and, as they passed by a water pump in the yard, she took Helen's hand and placed it underneath the pump and spelled out the word "w-a-t-e-r" again. This time something happened within Helen's brain. She saw the connection between the water and the word. Like an electric shock the conviction came that everything had a name, that everything was known, and that everything had importance, because it was loved. She went back into the house and tried to put the torn doll together. She determined that from now on life would be different, and it was.

Only the one who lives in the atmosphere of love can stand the strains of existence.

It is not the actual stresses of life so much that are responsible for our sorrows and our diseases, but our faulty reaction to those stresses.

You have heard of the two men who looked out through prison bars—one saw mud, and the other stars. That's the way it often is in life. Take retirement. One man retires, and he's having a grand time for he can do all the hobbies he has longed to do for years. His health thrives. But now take another man. He's no longer needed at the office. He's under his wife's feet at home. He sickens and dies. One condition for continuing to live is the conviction of usefulness. If you don't have this important conviction, life may draw to a sudden close. The feeling of uselessness is a negative feeling that is destructive.

The Australian aborigines have a ceremony called pointing the bone. The tribal leader points a bone at a person and, typically, the person will die within days. The reason why these aborigines have died is because of what has happened in the mind. It's how they interpreted the pointing of the bone that mattered. Because they believed the witchdoctor had the power to inflict death, as signaled by the bone pointing, they despaired and gave up the battle for life.

At the time of the second front in Europe, many allied soldiers were wounded on the Anzio beachhead. Strangely enough, only about a quarter as many of the wounded at Anzio called for morphine as would have called for it at home in local hospitals with the same amount of pain. Why? It was because the wounds at Anzio were a signal to the boys that they were going home. It meant they would soon be on the boat, and they would soon be with their families. To them the war would be over, and the wounds did not affect them as the same wounds would have affected them in civilian life.

Observe that while our health and happiness depends largely on what we eat and drink, they depend even more largely on what we think. What happens above your shoulders affects every cell of your body in every moment of time. It's safe for a ship to be in the sea, but it's not safe for the sea to be in the ship. Similarly, it's not the sorrows amidst which life's vessel plows that count, but whether those sorrows get inside the vessel. If we harbor trouble within the mind, we become ill. But if we believe that all things work together for good for those that love God, then even the gales of trouble will push us onwards to success and glory.

It is what is within us that determines the result of what happens to us. Here, the Christian has a tremendous advantage. Christ is in him, the hope of glory (Col 1:27). According to John 14-16, God has not left us alone, but has sent his Spirit to indwell us forever. That is the meaning of the Greek word for comforter—God sent alongside to help us in all circumstances. How that understanding changes life!

A mind that's filled with the promise of Scripture is a mind well fortified against the battering of daily experience. The apostle Peter advised us to "cast all your anxieties on him, for he cares about you" (1 Pet 5:7). In the letter to the Philippians, we find a recipe for successful living. We read in chapter 4: "Have no anxiety about anything, but in everything, by prayer and supplication, with thanksgiving, let your requests be known to God" (v.6). What a recipe! Be anxious about nothing, be prayerful for everything, and be thankful for anything. Try it, and keep trying it. Notice the result: "And the peace of God, which passes all understanding, will keep your hearts and your minds in Christ Jesus" (v. 7).

For Further Help

For evidence of the technical data endorsing the use of monounsaturates rather than a high carbohydrate diet consult the following:

New England Journal of Medicine, 1988, 319:829-34
Diabetes Care, 1994, xvii: 177-82; xvii: 311-5

These references support the positions taken by the writers, quoted in this book, who advocate monounsaturates as a primary therapy for type 2 diabetics.

For further information regarding how to control blood sugar by diet alone, see the following web page: http://www.lowcarblifestyle.com.

For poise of spirit and songs in the night, read often the following Scriptures: Psalms 23; 37; 62:5-8; 103; 142; Lamentations 3:19-26, 57; Isaiah 52:13 to 53:12; John 14:1-3; Romans. 8:28-39; 2 Corinthians 4:15-18; 12:8-10; Revelation 21; 22.

For a summary of that "good news" [the gospel], which "makes the heart to sing and the feet to dance," secure *Right with God Right Now*, by Desmond Ford.

Bibliography

Abrahamson, E. M. *Body, Mind, & Sugar.* New York: Avon Books, 1951.

Anderson, Linnea; Dibble, Marjorie V.; Turkki, Pirkko R.; Mitchell, Helen S.; Pynbergen, Henderika J. *Nutrition in Health and Disease,* 17th Edition. East Washington Square, Philadelphia: J.B. Lippincott, Company, 1982.

Atkins, Robert C. *Dr. Atkins' Age-Defying Diet Revolution.* New York: St. Martin's Press, 2000.

Bernstein, Richard K. *Dr. Bernstein's Diabetes Solution.* Little, Brown, and Company, 1997.

Biermann, June; Toohey, Barbara. *The Diabetic's Book.* Los Angeles: J.P. Tarcher, Inc., 1981.

Brandmiller, Jenny; Foster-Pawll, Kay; Colagiuri, Stephen; Leeds, Anthony. *The G.I. Factor.* Rydalmere, New South Wales, Australia: Hodder, reprinted 1998.

Burton, Benjamin T. *Human Nutrition,* 3rd Edition. H.J. Heinz Company, 1976.

Caliendo, Mary Alice. *Nutrition and Preventive Health Care.* New York: Macmillan Publishing Co., Inc., 1981.

Davidson, John K., M.D., Ph.D., ed. *Clinical Diabetes Mellitus.* New York, Stuttgart: Thieme, 2000.

Ezrin, Calvin; Kowalski, Robert E. *The Type 2 Diabetes Diet Book 3rd Edition.* Chicago: Lowell House, 1999.

Ford, Desmond. *Worth More Than a Million.* Desmond Ford Publications, 1990.

Ford, Desmond. *Stress and Distress.* Desmond Ford Publications, 1990.

Ford, Desmond. *How to Cope with Tragedy.* Desmond Ford Publications, 1990.

Ford, Desmond. *Right with God, Right Now.* Desmond Ford Publications, 1990.

See how to buy Desmond Ford's books on page 139.

Guthrie, Diana W.; Guthrie, Richard A. *The Diabetes Sourcebook.* Los Angeles: Lowell House, 1999.

Heller, Richard F.; Heller, Rachael F. *Healthy for Life.* New York: Penguin Books, USA, Inc., 1995.

Heller, Richard F.; Heller, Rachael F.; Vagnini, Frederic J. *The Carbohydrate Addict's Healthy Heart Program.* New York: Ballantine Books, 1999.

Herbert, Victor; Subak-Sharpe, Genell. *J. Total Nutrition*: The Only Guide You'll Ever Need. New York: St. Martin's Press, 1995.

Juliano, Joseph. *The Diabetic Male's Essential Guide to Living Well.* New York: Henry Holt and Company, 1998.

Krupp, Marcus A.; Schroeder, Steven A.; Tierney, Lawrence M., Jr. *Current Medical Diagnosis & Treatment, 1987.* Norwalk, Connecticut/Los Altos, California: Appleton & Lange, 1987.

Lodewick, Peter A., M.D.; Biermann, June; Toohey, Barbara. *The Diabetic Man.* Los Angeles, Lowell House, 1999.

Lodewick, Peter A., M.D. *A Diabetic Doctor Looks at Diabetes: His and Yours.* Pelham, Alabama: Southern Publishers Group, 1997.

Marshall, Charles W. *Vitamins and Minerals: Help or Harm?* Mt. Vernon: Consumers Union, 1985.

Murray, Michael. *Diabetes and Hypoglycemia.* Rocklin, Prima Publishing, 1994.

Norwood, Janet Worsley; Inlander Charles B. *Understanding Diabetes.* New York: Macmillan Company, 1999.

Pickup, John C.; Williams, Garth. *Textbook on Diabetes,* Blackwell Science, Inc., 1996.

Robin Eugene D., M.D. *Matters of Life and Death.* New York: W. H. Freeman and Company, 1984.

Robbins, John. *Diet for a New America,* Walpone, NH: Still Point Publishing, 1987.

Rosenfeld, Isadore. *The Best Treatment.* New York: Simon & Schuster, 1991.

Rubin, Alan L. *Diabetes for Dummies.* New York: IDG Books Worldwide, 1999.

Thrash, Agatha M., M.D.; Thrash, Calvin L., M.D. *Diabetes and the Hypoglycemic Syndrome.* Seale, AL: New Lifestyle Books, 1993.

Whitaker, Julian M., M.D. *Reversing Diabetes.* New York: Warner Books, Inc., 1987.

0-595-32779-6

41463048R00082

Made in the USA
Lexington, KY
14 May 2015